T0200291

# THE AMERICAN PSYCHIATRIC ASSOCIATION PRACTICE GUIDELINE ON THE USE OF Antipsychotics TO Treat Agitation OR Psychosis IN Patients WITH Dementia

## Guideline Writing Group

Victor I. Reus, M.D., *Chair*
Laura J. Fochtmann, M.D., M.B.I., *Vice-Chair*
A. Evan Eyler, M.D., M.P.H.
Donald M. Hilty, M.D.
Marcela Horvitz-Lennon, M.D., M.P.H.
Michael D. Jibson, Ph.D., M.D.
Oscar L. Lopez, M.D.
Jane Mahoney, Ph.D., R.N., PMHCNS-BC
Jagoda Pasic, M.D., Ph.D.
Zaldy S. Tan, M.D., M.P.H.
Cheryl D. Wills, M.D.

## Systematic Review Group

Laura J. Fochtmann, M.D., M.B.I.
Richard Rhoads, M.D.
Joel Yager, M.D.

## APA Steering Committee on Practice Guidelines

Michael J. Vergare, M.D., *Chair*
Daniel J. Anzia, M.D., *Vice-Chair*
Thomas J. Craig, M.D.
Deborah Cowley, M.D.
Nassir Ghaemi, M.D., M.P.H.
David A. Kahn, M.D.
John M. Oldham, M.D.
Carlos N. Pato, M.D., Ph.D.
Mary S. Sciutto, M.D.

## Assembly Liaisons

John P.D. Shemo, M.D., *Chair of Area Liaisons*
John M. de Figueiredo, M.D.
Marvin Koss, M.D.
William M. Greenberg, M.D.
Bhasker Dave, M.D.
Robert M. McCarron, D.O.
Jason W. Hunziker, M.D.

APA wishes to acknowledge the contributions of APA staff (Seung-Hee Hong, Karen Kanefield, Kristin Kroeger Pta-kowski, and Samantha Shugarman, M.S.) and former APA staff (Robert Kunkle, M.A.). APA and the Guideline Writing Group especially thank Laura J. Fochtmann, M.D., M.B.I., Seung-Hee Hong, and Robert Kunkle, M.A., for their outstand-ing work and effort on developing this guideline. APA also thanks the APA Steering Committee on Practice Guidelines (Michael Vergare, M.D., Chair), liaisons from the APA Assembly for their input and assistance, and APA Councils and others for providing feedback during the comment period. Thanks also go to those individuals who completed the Expert Consensus Survey.

The authors have worked to ensure that all information in this book concerning drug dosages, schedules, and routes of administration is accurate as of the time of publication and consistent with standards set by the U.S. Food and Drug Administration and the general medical community. As medical research and practice advance, however, therapeutic standards may change. For this reason and because human and mechanical errors sometimes occur, we recommend that readers follow the advice of a physician who is directly involved in their care or the care of a member of their family.

For inquiries about permissions or licensing, please contact Permissions & Licensing, American Psychiatric Publishing, 1000 Wilson Boulevard, Suite 1825, Arlington, VA 22209-3901 or submit inquiries online at: http://www.appi.org/CustomerService/Pages/Permissions.aspx.

If you wish to buy 50 or more copies of the same title, please go to www.appi.org/specialdiscounts for more information.

Manufactured in the United States of America on acid-free paper
20  19  18  17  16     5  4  3  2  1
First Edition

American Psychiatric Association
1000 Wilson Boulevard
Arlington, VA 22209-3901
www.psych.org

ISBN-13: 978-0-89042-677-7

**Library of Congress Cataloging-in-Publication Data**
A CIP record is available from the Library of Congress.

**British Library Cataloguing in Publication Data**
A CIP record is available from the British Library.

# Contents

# Acronyms/Abbreviations

**ABPN**  American Board of Psychiatry and Neurology

**ACCME**  Accreditation Council for Continuing Medical Education

**AD**  Alzheimer's disease

**AHRQ**  Agency for Healthcare Research and Quality

**AIMS**  Abnormal Involuntary Movement Scale

**APA**  American Psychiatric Association

**BEHAVE-AD**  Behavioral Pathology in Alzheimer's Disease

**BMI**  Body mass index

**BPRS**  Brief Psychiatric Rating Scale

**BPSD**  Behavioral and psychological symptoms of dementia

**CATIE-AD**  Clinical Antipsychotic Trials of Intervention Effectiveness for Alzheimer's Disease

**CGI**  Clinical Global Impressions

**CGI-C**  Clinical Global Impression of Change

**CI**  Confidence interval

**CMAI**  Cohen-Mansfield Agitation Inventory

**CVA**  Cerebrovascular accident

**DLB**  Dementia with Lewy body

**DSM-IV**  *Diagnostic and Statistical Manual of Mental Disorders*, 4th Edition

**DSM-5**  *Diagnostic and Statistical Manual of Mental Disorders*, 5th Edition

**EPS**  Extrapyramidal symptoms

**FAST**  Functional assessment staging

**FGA**  First-generation antipsychotic

**GRADE**  Grading of Recommendations Assessment, Development and Evaluation

**HR**  Hazard ratio

**ICD-10**  *International Classification of Diseases*, 10th Revision

**IR**  Immediate release

**IRR**  Incidence rate ratio

**ITT**  Intention to treat

**MDS**  Minimum data set

**MI**  Myocardial infarction

**MMSE**  Mini-Mental State Examination

**NC**  Not calculated

**NIA**  National Institute on Aging

**NIMH**  National Institute of Mental Health

**NINCDS/ADRDA**  National Institute of Neurological and Communicative Diseases and Stroke/Alzheimer's Disease and Related Disorders Association

**NNH**  Number needed to harm

**NPI**  Neuropsychiatric Inventory

**NPI-NH** or **NPI/NH**  Neuropsychiatric Inventory—Nursing Home

**NPI-Q**  Neuropsychiatric Inventory Questionnaire

**NQF**  National Quality Forum

**NS**  Not significant

**OR**  Odds ratio

**PANSS-EC**  Positive and Negative Symptom Scale—Excitement Component

**PICOTS**  Patient population, Intervention, Comparator, Outcome, Timing, Setting

**QTc**  Corrected QT interval

**RCT**  Randomized controlled trial

**RR**  Rate ratio

**SAS**  Simpson-Angus Scale

**SD**  Standard deviation

**SGA**  Second-generation antipsychotic

**SIB**  Severe Impairment Battery

**SMD**  Standardized mean difference

**TD**  Tardive dyskinesia

**TIA**  Transient ischemic attack

**VTE**  Venous thromboembolism

**XR**  Extended release

# Introduction

## Overview of the Development Process

Since the publication of the Institute of Medicine (2011) report *Clinical Practice Guidelines We Can Trust*, there has been an increasing focus on using clearly defined, transparent processes for rating the quality of evidence and the strength of the overall body of evidence in systematic reviews of the scientific literature. This guideline was developed using a process intended to be consistent with the recommendations of the Institute of Medicine (2011), the Principles for the Development of Specialty Society Clinical Guidelines of the Council of Medical Specialty Societies (2012), and the requirements of the Agency for Healthcare Research and Quality (AHRQ) for inclusion of a guideline in the National Guideline Clearinghouse. Parameters used for the guideline's systematic review are included with the full text of the guideline; the development process is fully described in a document available on the American Psychiatric Association (APA) website (http://www.psychiatry.org/File%20Library/Psychiatrists/Practice/Clinical%20Practice%20Guidelines/Guideline-Development-Process.pdf). To supplement the expertise of members of the guideline work group, we used a "snowball" survey methodology (Yager et al. 2014) to identify experts on the treatment of agitation or psychosis in individuals with dementia. Results of this expert survey are included in Appendix B of the practice guideline.

## Rating the Strength of Research Evidence and Recommendations

The guideline recommendations are rated using GRADE (Grading of Recommendations Assessment, Development and Evaluation), which is used by multiple professional organizations around the world to develop practice guideline recommendations (Guyatt et al. 2013). With the GRADE approach, the strength of a guideline statement reflects the level of confidence that potential benefits of an intervention outweigh the potential harms (Andrews et al. 2013). This level of confidence is informed by available evidence, which includes evidence from clinical trials as well as expert opinion and patient values and preferences. Evidence for the benefit of a particular intervention within a specific clinical context is identified through systematic review and is then balanced against the evidence for harms. In this regard, harms are broadly defined and might include direct and indirect costs of the intervention (including opportunity costs) as well as potential for adverse effects from the intervention. Whenever possible, we have followed the admonition to current guideline development groups to avoid using words such as "might" or "consider" in drafting these recommendations because they can be difficult for clinicians to interpret (Shiffman et al. 2005).

As described under "Guideline Development Process," each final rating is a consensus judgment of the authors of the guideline and is endorsed by the APA Board of Trustees. A "recommendation" (denoted by the numeral 1 after the guideline statement) indicates confidence that the benefits of the intervention clearly outweigh the harms. A "suggestion" (denoted by the numeral 2 after the guideline statement) indicates uncertainty (i.e., the balance of benefits and harms is difficult to judge, or either the benefits or the harms are unclear). Each guideline statement also has an associated rating for the "strength of supporting research evidence." Three ratings are used—high, moderate, and low (denoted by the letters A, B, and C, respectively)—and reflect the level of confidence that the evidence for a guideline statement reflects a true effect based on consistency of findings across studies, directness of the effect on a specific health outcome, and precision of the estimate of effect and risk of bias in available studies (Agency for Healthcare Research and Quality 2014; Balshem et al. 2011; Guyatt et al. 2006).

It is well recognized that there are guideline topics and clinical circumstances for which high-quality evidence from clinical trials is not possible or is unethical to obtain (Council of Medical Specialty Societies 2012). For example, many questions need to be asked as part of an assessment, and inquiring about a particular symptom or element of the history cannot be separated out for study as a discrete intervention. It would also be impossible to separate changes in outcome due to assessment from changes in outcomes due to ensuing treatment. Research on psychiatric assessments and some psychiatric interventions can also be complicated by multiple confounding factors such as the interaction between the clinician and the patient or the patient's unique circumstances and experiences. For these and other reasons, many topics covered in this guideline have relied on forms of evidence such as consensus opinions of experienced clinicians or indirect findings from observational studies rather than being based on research from randomized trials. The GRADE working group and guidelines developed by other professional organizations have noted that a strong recommendation may be appropriate even in the absence of research evidence when sensible alternatives do not exist (Andrews et al. 2013; Brito et al. 2013; Djulbegovic et al. 2009; Hazlehurst et al. 2013).

# Proper Use of Guidelines

The APA Practice Guidelines are assessments of current scientific and clinical information provided as an educational service. The guidelines 1) should not be considered as a statement of the standard of care or inclusive of all proper treatments or methods of care; 2) are not continually updated and may not reflect the most recent evidence, as new evidence may emerge between the time information is developed and when the guidelines are published or read; 3) address only the question(s) or issue(s) specifically identified; 4) do not mandate any particular course of medical care; 5) are not intended to substitute for the independent professional judgment of the treating provider; and 6) do not account for individual variation among patients. As such, it is not possible to draw conclusions about the effects of omitting a particular recommendation, either in general or for a specific patient. Furthermore, adherence to these guidelines will not ensure a successful outcome for every individual, nor should these guidelines be interpreted as including all proper methods of evaluation and care or excluding other acceptable methods of evaluation and care aimed at the same results. The ultimate recommendation regarding a particular assessment, clinical procedure, or treatment plan must be made by the clinician in light of the psychiatric evaluation, other clinical data, and the diagnostic and treatment options available. Such recommendations should be made in collaboration with the patient, whenever possible, and incorporate the patient's personal and sociocultural preferences and values in order to enhance the therapeutic alliance, adherence to treatment, and treatment outcomes. For all of these reasons, APA cautions against the use of guidelines in litigation. Use of these guidelines is voluntary. APA provides the guidelines on an "as is" basis and makes no warranty, expressed or implied, regarding them. APA assumes no responsibility for any injury or damage to persons or property arising out of or related to any use of the guidelines or for any errors or omissions.

# Guidelines and Implementation

## Guideline Statements

### Assessment of Behavioral/Psychological Symptoms of Dementia

**Statement 1.** APA recommends that patients with dementia[1] be assessed for the type, frequency, severity, pattern, and timing of symptoms. **(1C)**

**Statement 2.** APA recommends that patients with dementia be assessed for pain and other potentially modifiable contributors to symptoms as well as for factors, such as the subtype of dementia, that may influence choices of treatment. **(1C)**

**Statement 3.** APA recommends that in patients with dementia with agitation or psychosis, response to treatment be assessed with a quantitative measure. **(1C)**

### Development of a Comprehensive Treatment Plan

**Statement 4.** APA recommends that patients with dementia have a documented comprehensive treatment plan that includes appropriate person-centered nonpharmacological and pharmacological interventions, as indicated. **(1C)**

### Assessment of Benefits and Risks of Antipsychotic Treatment for the Patient

**Statement 5.** APA recommends that nonemergency antipsychotic medication should only be used for the treatment of agitation or psychosis in patients with dementia when symptoms are severe, are dangerous, and/or cause significant distress to the patient. **(1B)**

**Statement 6.** APA recommends reviewing the clinical response to nonpharmacological interventions prior to nonemergency use of an antipsychotic medication to treat agitation or psychosis in patients with dementia. **(1C)**

**Statement 7.** APA recommends that before nonemergency treatment with an antipsychotic is initiated in patients with dementia, the potential risks and benefits from antipsychotic medication be assessed by the clinician and discussed with the patient (if clinically feasible) as well as with the patient's surrogate decision maker (if relevant) with input from family or others involved with the patient. **(1C)**

---

[1]Throughout this guideline, we use the term *dementia*, which was used in the evidence that was considered in developing these recommendations. These recommendations are also meant to apply to individuals with major neurocognitive disorder, as defined in the APA's *Diagnostic and Statistical Manual of Mental Disorders, 5th Edition* (DSM-5).

# Dosing, Duration, and Monitoring of Antipsychotic Treatment

**Statement 8.** APA recommends that if a risk/benefit assessment favors the use of an antipsychotic for behavioral/psychological symptoms in patients with dementia, treatment should be initiated at a low dose to be titrated up to the minimum effective dose as tolerated. **(1B)**

**Statement 9.** APA recommends that if a patient with dementia experiences a clinically significant side effect of antipsychotic treatment, the potential risks and benefits of antipsychotic medication should be reviewed by the clinician to determine if tapering and discontinuing of the medication is indicated. **(1C)**

**Statement 10.** APA recommends that in patients with dementia with agitation or psychosis, if there is no clinically significant response after a 4-week trial of an adequate dose of an antipsychotic drug, the medication should be tapered and withdrawn. **(1B)**

**Statement 11.** APA recommends that in a patient who has shown a positive response to treatment, decision making about possible tapering of antipsychotic medication should be accompanied by a discussion with the patient (if clinically feasible) as well as with the patient's surrogate decision maker (if relevant) with input from family or others involved with the patient. The aim of such a discussion is to elicit their preferences and concerns and to review the initial goals, observed benefits and side effects of antipsychotic treatment, and potential risks of continued exposure to antipsychotics, as well as past experience with antipsychotic medication trials and tapering attempts. **(1C)**

**Statement 12.** APA recommends that in patients with dementia who show adequate response of behavioral/psychological symptoms to treatment with an antipsychotic drug, an attempt to taper and withdraw the drug should be made within 4 months of initiation, unless the patient experienced a recurrence of symptoms with prior attempts at tapering of antipsychotic medication. **(1C)**

**Statement 13.** APA recommends that in patients with dementia whose antipsychotic medication is being tapered, assessment of symptoms should occur at least monthly during the taper and for at least 4 months after medication discontinuation to identify signs of recurrence and trigger a reassessment of the benefits and risks of antipsychotic treatment. **(1C)**

# Use of Specific Antipsychotic Medications, Depending on Clinical Context

**Statement 14.** APA recommends that in the absence of delirium, if nonemergency antipsychotic medication treatment is indicated, haloperidol should not be used as a first-line agent. **(1B)**

**Statement 15.** APA recommends that in patients with dementia with agitation or psychosis, a long-acting injectable antipsychotic medication should not be utilized unless it is otherwise indicated for a co-occurring chronic psychotic disorder. **(1B)**

# Rationale

The goal of this guideline is to improve the care of patients with dementia who are exhibiting agitation or psychosis. More specifically, this guideline focuses on the judicious use of antipsychotic medications when agitation or psychosis occurs in association with dementia and does not review evidence for or focus on other pharmacological interventions. The guideline is intended to apply to individuals with dementia in all settings of care as well as to care delivered by generalist and specialist clinicians. Recommendations regarding treatment with antipsychotic medications are not intended to apply to individuals who are receiving antipsychotic medication for another indication (e.g., chronic psychotic illness) or individuals who are receiving an antipsychotic medication in an urgent context.

A practice guideline for this subject is needed because of the prevalence of dementia in the older adult population, the common occurrence of agitation and psychotic symptoms among patients with dementia, the variability in current treatment practices, and the risks associated with some forms of treatment.

Globally, dementia is associated with a sizeable public health burden that is growing rapidly as the population ages (Brookmeyer et al. 2007; Sloane et al. 2002; World Health Organization 2012). The burden on caregivers is also substantial and is increased when dementia is associated with behavioral and psychological symptoms and particularly with agitation or aggression (Dauphinot et al. 2015; Ornstein and Gaugler 2012; Thyrian et al. 2015).

Estimates suggest that 5%–10% of individuals over age 65 and 30%–40% of individuals over age 85 in the United States have dementia (Ferri et al. 2005; Hebert et al. 2013; Prince et al. 2013). Data from a nationally representative sample suggested that in 2002 approximately 3.4 million individuals had dementia; Alzheimer's disease was present in about three-quarters of these individuals (Plassman et al. 2007). A later study in an urban community sample estimated that 4.7 million individuals age 65 years or older had Alzheimer's disease dementia as of 2010 (Hebert et al. 2013), but this figure likely includes individuals with mixed types of dementia as well as Alzheimer's disease dementia (Plassman et al. 2007; Wilson et al. 2011).

In addition to cognitive impairments, individuals with dementia often come to clinical attention because of symptoms of a behavioral disturbance (e.g., irritability, agitation, aggression) or psychosis. Many people who experience these symptoms become distressed or dangerous to self or others, but some do not. The frequency of such behavioral and psychological symptoms in dementia varies with the clinical setting and severity of dementia as well as with the study design. In population-based samples, the point prevalence of delusions was 18%–25%, with hallucinations in 10%–15% and agitation or aggression in 9%–30% of individuals studied (Lyketsos et al. 2000, 2002; Savva et al. 2009). In about half of individuals, these symptoms were rated as severe in frequency, severity, and/or associated distress (Lyketsos et al. 2002).

A systematic review of psychotic symptoms among persons with Alzheimer's disease across different settings of care found median prevalences for psychosis of 41.1% (range 12.2%–74.1%), 18% (range 4%–41%) for hallucinations, 36% (range 9.3%–63%) for delusions, and 25.6% (range 3.6%–38.9%) for other psychotic symptoms such as misidentification (Ropacki and Jeste 2005). In nursing home settings, another systematic review (Selbæk et al. 2013) found that delusions were present in 22% (range 1%–54%) of individuals, with hallucinations in 14% (range 1%–39%). Delusions and hallucinations persisted in 13%–66% and 25%–100% of study subjects, respectively. At least one symptom of agitation was present in 79% of nursing home subjects (range 66%–83%), with aggressive behaviors noted in 32% (range 11%–77%) and other signs of agitation in 36% (range 17%–67%). Agitation and aggression were persistent in 53%–75% of individuals. Thus, an overwhelming majority of older adults with dementia will develop psychosis or agitation during the course of their illness. Furthermore, these symptoms are often persistent, occur with increasing frequency as cognition became more impaired, and are more prevalent among residents of nursing home or inpatient facilities as compared with community settings (Lyketsos et al. 2002; Ropacki and Jeste 2005; Savva et al. 2009; Selbæk et al. 2013; Steinberg et al. 2008).

Treatment of psychotic symptoms and agitation in individuals with dementia has often involved use of antipsychotic medications. In recent years, the risks associated with use of these agents in the older adult population have become apparent (see sections "Potential Benefits and Harms" and "Review of Supporting Research Evidence" [Appendix A] in this guideline). The need to develop guidelines for appropriate use of antipsychotic medications in patients with dementia follows from this evidence base.

# Potential Benefits and Harms

## Benefits

In individuals with dementia, as in any patient who presents with a psychiatric symptom, an initial assessment serves as a foundation for further evaluation and treatment planning (American Psychiatric Association 2015b). Assessing the type, frequency, severity, pattern, and timing of symptoms such as agitation and psychosis can help in identifying possible contributors and in targeting interventions to address symptoms and their causes. Pain is a common contributor to agitation or aggression and may signal other physical conditions, which may also need intervention. It is similarly important to determine the subtype(s) of dementia that is present, as this has implications for treating behavioral/psychological symptoms as well as providing information on likely disease course. The initial assessment also provides baseline information on symptoms, which is relevant to tracking of symptom progression or effects of intervention. Use of a quantitative measure to document information on symptoms in a systematic fashion can be helpful in monitoring the patient's progress and assessing effects of treatment. A comprehensive treatment plan, as an outgrowth of the initial assessment, is beneficial in fostering a thorough review of the patient's clinical presentation and in reviewing potential options for care that are person-centered and aimed at improving overall quality of life. Discussing the benefits and risks of possible treatments with the patient and surrogate decision makers is valuable in engaging them and helping them make informed decisions. Such discussions can also be beneficial by providing education on dementia and its symptoms and on available therapeutic options.

There are a number of potential advantages to including nonpharmacological interventions as a part of a comprehensive treatment plan. The most consistently effective interventions have focused on home-based caregivers and aim to develop their skills, improve their general well-being, and reduce their perceived burden (Adelman et al. 2014; Kales et al. 2015). These caregiver-related outcomes are predictive of whether a dementia patient is able to remain in the community or will be transitioned to institutional care (de Vugt et al. 2005; Miller et al. 2012). Other interventions can help in improving the culture and safety of the care environment and in conveying to patients and families that their needs and comfort are important. For most behavioral interventions there have not been a sufficient number of large-scale, well-controlled studies from which to draw conclusions about efficacy or safety in treating agitation or psychosis (Brasure et al. 2016). When studies with less rigorous designs and a broader range of target symptoms are also considered, modest benefits of behavioral interventions have been found (Brodaty and Arasaratnam 2012; Kales et al. 2015; Livingston et al. 2014). Among the specific benefits reported are reductions in agitation and aggression, alleviation of depression, improvement in sleep, and increased constructive activity. Studies of environmental modifications are even more limited than studies of behavioral interventions, and available data from clinical trials do not show significant effects (Kong et al. 2009). Nevertheless, anecdotal observations suggest that some individuals with dementia may benefit from reducing environmental clutter and ambient noise, optimizing lighting and walkways, providing cues to heighten orientation, and other environmental modifications.

Placebo-controlled trials of nonantipsychotic medications have not been reviewed in this practice guideline, and, thus, no recommendations are made about the appropriateness or sequence of their use based on their benefits and harms. In addition, no conclusions can be drawn from head-to-head comparisons between nonantipsychotic drugs (e.g., antidepressants, cholinesterase inhibitors, memantine) and antipsychotic drugs because of insufficient evidence (see "Review of Supporting Research Evidence" in Appendix A).

Expert consensus suggests that use of an antipsychotic medication in individuals with dementia can be appropriate, particularly in individuals with dangerous agitation or psychosis (see "Expert Opinion Survey Data: Results" in Appendix B), and can minimize the risk of violence, reduce patient distress, improve the patient's quality of life, and reduce caregiver burden. However, in clinical trials, the benefits of antipsychotic medications are at best small (Corbett et al. 2014; Kales et al. 2015; see "Review of Supporting Research Evidence" in Appendix A) whether assessed through placebo-controlled trials, head-to-head comparison trials, or discontinuation trials. Effect sizes of second-generation antipsychotics (SGAs) range from nonsignificant to small depending on symptom domain (agitation, psychosis, and overall behavioral/psychological symptoms) and agent (see "Review of Supporting Research Evidence" in Appendix A). First-generation antipsychotics (FGAs) are deemed not different from SGAs in the management of agitation and overall behavioral/psychological symptoms, but the strength of the evidence for the comparisons is low, and haloperidol is the predominant agent that has been studied. There is not enough evidence to compare the effects of FGAs and SGAs on psychosis.

On the basis of both strength of the research evidence and effect size (moderate and small, respectively), the best evidence for SGA efficacy is in treatment of agitation, results that are driven by findings with risperidone treatment. Although evidence for the efficacy of SGAs suggests low utility (low strength of evidence for a very small effect) in the management of psychosis, the evidence for risperidone is substantially better than for the class (moderate strength of evidence for a small effect). Likewise, the efficacy evidence for SGAs in the management of overall behavioral/psychological symptoms also suggests low utility (high strength of evidence for a very small effect); the evidence for aripiprazole is substantially better than for the class (moderate strength of evidence for a small effect). For patients receiving treatment with an SGA as compared with placebo in the Clinical Antipsychotic Trials of Intervention Effectiveness for Alzheimer's Disease (CATIE-AD), a modest reduction in caregiver burden was noted (Mohamed et al. 2012).

A number of studies have assessed the effects of discontinuing an antipsychotic medication in subjects with dementia, and the findings suggest a small effect of antipsychotic treatment. In individuals receiving placebo, there was a higher likelihood of symptom recurrence as compared with those continuing to receive an antipsychotic (moderate confidence), with some post hoc analyses showing that individuals who had higher baseline levels of symptoms or who were taking higher baseline doses of antipsychotic were more likely to have recurrent symptoms with discontinuation (Declercq et al. 2013; see "Review of Supporting Research Evidence" in Appendix A).

A dose-response effect, if present, can also provide suggestive evidence for a therapeutic benefit of a medication. The absence of a dose-response relationship is less informative; studies in which a dose-response relationship is absent are often underpowered, and a sufficiently wide range of doses is not always tested. Five published randomized controlled trials (RCTs) assessed differing doses of antipsychotic medications in managing behavioral and psychological symptoms of dementia, but these studies were of varying quality, had inconsistent findings, and often showed no therapeutic benefit at the highest dose (see "Review of Supporting Research Evidence" in Appendix A). There are no published studies on the optimal duration of antipsychotic treatment in individuals with dementia, and experts are divided in their opinion on optimal treatment duration (see "Expert Opinion Survey Data: Results" in Appendix B).

## Harms

No studies have directly assessed harm from conducting an assessment or developing a comprehensive treatment plan. It is possible that questioning during an assessment may be upsetting to some patients and could increase rather than reduce agitation. Such worsening of symptoms is expected to be brief because the clinician will be able to curtail questioning or adjust the interview style and format to the patient's responses. In an emergent situation, harm could result to the patient or others if interventions are delayed in order to complete assessment, treatment plan documentation, or discussions with the patient, family, or surrogate decision makers.

None of the available studies have reported direct harm to patients from behavioral interventions (Ayalon et al. 2006; Brasure et al. 2016). Reported risks associated with these interventions include falls and orthopedic injuries during physical activity, or worsening agitation and aggression with some approaches, particularly those involving physical contact between caregiver and patient (e.g., massage). Harm could also result to the patient or others if emergency interventions were to be delayed to complete trials of behavioral treatments. No direct comparisons of risk between behavioral and pharmacological therapies have been reported. No data are available on harms of environmental modifications or other nonpharmacological interventions, but again, the potential for harm is likely to be quite small.

With antipsychotic medications, the drugs' potential for harms must be balanced against their modest evidence of benefit. As with any drug, this requires assessing the benefits and harms of prescribing the drug for an individual patient. No studies are available that assess the harms of withholding or delaying a trial of antipsychotic medication for individuals with agitation or psychosis in association with dementia. However, clinical observations suggest that such delays could lead to poorer outcomes for some individuals, such as physical injury to themselves or others, disruptions of relationships with family or other caregivers, or loss of housing due to unmanageable behavioral and psychological symptoms.

This estimation of benefits and risks should also consider clinical characteristics of the patient. For example, patients with Lewy body dementia or Parkinson's disease dementia are at increased risk for adverse effects, which are typically more severe than in patients with other types of dementia and in some instances have been associated with irreversible cognitive decompensation or death. The risk of adverse effects may also be influenced by a history of falls or the presence of co-occurring medical conditions such as other neurological conditions, hypotension, diabetes, or cardiac or cerebrovascular disease.

The strength of evidence for harms of antipsychotic agents ranges from insufficient to high depending on the specific adverse effect; however, on the whole, there is consistent evidence that antipsychotics are associated with clinically significant adverse effects, including mortality (see section "Review of Supporting Research Evidence" in Appendix A). Harms data are rarely a primary outcome of randomized trials, and there is a paucity of randomized head-to-head comparisons of antipsychotic medications using equivalent doses of drug. In addition, the absolute number of serious adverse events in randomized trials is typically small, and this confounds statistical analysis. For example, pooled data from randomized placebo-controlled trials (Maglione et al. 2011) showed deaths in 8 of 340 (2.4%) individuals treated with aripiprazole as compared with 3 of 253 (1.2%) receiving placebo (pooled odds ratio [OR]=2.37 from three studies; $P$=not significant [NS]), 2 of 278 (0.7%) treated with olanzapine as compared with 4 of 232 (1.7%) receiving placebo (pooled OR = 0.48 from two studies; $P$=NS), 5 of 185 (2.7%) treated with quetiapine as compared with 7 of 241 (2.9%) receiving placebo (pooled OR=0.91 from two studies; $P$=NS), and 39 of 1,561 (2.5%) treated with risperidone as compared with 17 of 916 (1.9%) receiving placebo (pooled OR=1.19; $P$=NS). For SGAs as a group, meta-analysis of the data from randomized placebo-controlled trials indicates that there is a statistically significant increase in mortality relative to placebo (Schneider et al. 2005).

From a methodological standpoint, data on harms generally come from studies that are less rigorous than randomized trials, such as observational or cohort studies. Administrative database studies are increasingly common and track associations between prescribed medications and diagnoses. This research cannot consider the effects of confounding variables such as dementia severity, co-occurring conditions, or the magnitude of agitation or psychosis. Nevertheless, administrative databases do permit study of large patient samples, which is important when looking at infrequent events. Some of these naturalistic studies have suggested a heightened risk of treatment with haloperidol and other FGAs and possible differences in risk among the other antipsychotic medications (see section "Review of Supporting Research Evidence" in Appendix A). However, as with studies of antipsychotic benefits, the limitations of existing research make it difficult to draw precise conclusions about the likely harms of treatment for an individual patient.

In addition to mortality, other serious adverse events of antipsychotic medications in individuals with dementia have been reported, including stroke, acute cardiovascular events, metabolic effects, and pulmonary effects (see section "Review of Supporting Research Evidence" in Appendix A). The strength of the evidence is low for stroke, but pooled analyses for risperidone and olanzapine suggest an increase in risk relative to placebo. The strength of the evidence on acute cardiovascular events is also low; however, there is some evidence of increased risk for all antipsychotics, with the risk being highest early in the treatment, and of a greater risk with risperidone and olanzapine than with other agents. Although the evidence on metabolic effects of antipsychotics (including weight gain, diabetes, dyslipidemia, and metabolic syndrome) is not as strong in individuals with dementia as it is in younger adults, the existing evidence is in keeping with what is largely known about this risk: highest for olanzapine and risperidone and lowest for aripiprazole and high-potency FGAs. Antipsychotic treatment in individuals with dementia also appears to carry an increased risk for pneumonia and for venous thromboembolism, but the strength of this evidence is low, with no apparent difference between FGAs and SGAs. Evidence is variable for other adverse effects, including cognitive worsening, sedation/fatigue, anticholinergic effects, postural hypotension, prolonged QTc intervals, sexual dysfunction, and extrapyramidal symptoms (e.g., parkinsonism, dystonia, tardive dyskinesia). However, case reports and observational data suggest a substantial increase in the likelihood of adverse effects when individuals with Lewy body dementia or Parkinson's disease dementia receive antipsychotic treatment (Aarsland et al. 2005; Stinton et al. 2015). In some instances, these adverse effects have included irreversible cognitive decompensation or death. Less information is available for individuals with frontotemporal lobar degeneration, but a heightened sensitivity to antipsychotic medications has also been reported (Pijnenburg et al. 2003). No evidence is available that specifically addresses the possible harms of antipsychotic treatment in individuals being treated for chronic psychotic illness who subsequently develop dementia.

In terms of decisions about doses of antipsychotic medications, there is strong evidence that SGAs are associated with clinically significant dose-related adverse effects (Maust et al. 2015; see section "Review of Supporting Research Evidence" in Appendix A). Thus, if medications are begun at a low dose and increased gradually depending on clinical response, adverse effects may be minimized. On the other hand, it is possible that harms to the patient or others may occur if the response to treatment is delayed by underdosing of medication, particularly in emergency situations.

In terms of optimal treatment duration, the data suggest that the greatest risk of mortality occurs in the initial 120 days of antipsychotic use (Maust et al. 2015; see section "Review of Supporting Research Evidence" in Appendix A). The mechanisms by which heightened mortality could occur are unclear. In observational studies, unmeasured predisposing factors may lead both to a greater likelihood of antipsychotic treatment and to heightened mortality. However, although the greatest period of risk appears to occur with treatment initiation, the risk of adverse effects also persists with longer-term treatment. The cut-point of 120 days is, at least partially, an artifact of the designs of available research. Discontinuation studies suggest that antipsychotic medications can be tapered and stopped in many patients without return of symptoms (see section "Review of Supporting Research Evidence" in Appendix A). Expert consensus also suggests that an attempt at tapering an antipsychotic medication is indicated (see section "Expert Opinion Survey Data: Results" in Appendix B), with variation in the suggested timing of a taper attempt; however, only a small fraction of experts favored maintaining the dose of medication without a specific target date for a tapering attempt. Although some individuals will have recurrence of symptoms with antipsychotic discontinuation (moderate confidence), such risks can likely be mitigated by careful monitoring during treatment cessation with adjustments made in the medication tapering plan based on clinical response. However, there are no data on the most appropriate frequency for monitoring or the extent to which monitoring can reduce the severity or risk of symptom recurrence, which is unpredictable. There is insufficient evidence to determine whether individuals with more severe dementia, psychosis, or agitation will have a greater risk of symptom recurrence with discontinuation. There are also no data on whether symptom response is equivalent if antipsychotic medication is resumed after recurrence of symptoms.

No studies have examined the use of long-acting injectable antipsychotic medications in individuals with dementia. However, the longer duration of action of these medications suggests that they would be associated with an increased risk of harm relative to oral formulations or short-acting parenteral formulations of antipsychotic medications, particularly in frail elders.

## Costs

The costs of assessment, treatment planning, and discussions with patients, family, or other surrogate decision makers relate to clinician time. Discussions with family or surrogate decision makers can also introduce direct or indirect costs to those individuals (e.g., lost work time, transportation). The feasibility of any treatment must also consider the unique situation of the patient and family, such as access to transportation, insurance status and coverage for specific services, and the effects of treatment requirements on the caregiver's time or employment.

A small number of studies on the cost-effectiveness of behavioral treatments have consistently shown modest but favorable results for specific interventions (Gitlin et al. 2010). Prospective cost estimates for specific patients must take into account the need for individual therapists, the number and duration of required sessions, and the costs of home visits for community-based interventions (Brodaty and Arasaratnam 2012). Typically, such expenses have been assessed in terms of increased patient activities in the same setting and associated increases in personnel-related costs, but have not been weighed against the cost of pharmacological interventions, the cost of institutionalization for patients who cannot be managed at home or in less restrictive settings, or the cost of injuries to patients and caregivers during episodes of agitated or aggressive behavior.

The CATIE-AD trial (Rosenheck et al. 2007) examined the cost-effectiveness of antipsychotic treatment for outpatients with Alzheimer's disease and psychosis, aggression, or agitation. Although individuals treated with an SGA showed no difference in quality adjusted life years or functional measures as compared with individuals receiving placebo, there were significantly lower costs in the placebo group. However, with the availability of generic SGAs, the costs of medication are likely to be less. We are not aware of studies on the cost-effectiveness of antipsychotic treatment for individuals with dementia in inpatient or nursing facilities or for severely agitated or aggressive individuals who require constant supervision.

## Balancing of Benefits and Harms in Rating the Strength of Recommendations

Consensus on rating the strength of recommendations was high within the guideline writing group, and the statements were recommended unanimously. One group member (O.L.L.) chose not to vote on statements 7–15. The results of the expert opinion survey and input from the Alzheimer's Association were incorporated in decisions about benefits and harms as noted below. Because costs of medications and other interventions vary widely, the guideline writing group did not consider cost-related considerations in weighing the benefits and harms of recommendations.

The strength of research evidence supporting these guideline statements is low to moderate. Statements 1, 2, 3, 4, 6, 7, 9, 11, and 13 are based on expert consensus that is derived from fundamental and generally accepted principles of medical ethics and medical practice, including elements of conducting an assessment, reviewing responses to prior treatments, and developing a plan of treatment. These statements also emphasize the importance of involving patients and surrogate decision makers, with input from family members and others. Perspectives of patients and their care partners highlight the need for such discussions and input at all steps of the decision-making and treatment-monitoring process to identify person-centered goals, values, and preferences that can shape care and enhance outcomes.

In statements 4 and 6, which address treatment planning and review of response to nonpharmacological interventions, the group chose not to comment on specific psychopharmacological medications other than antipsychotic medications. Although the guideline writing group only reviewed evidence on antipsychotic medications during the development process, available systematic reviews suggested that the harms of nonpharmacological interventions were minimal. In contrast, with other pharmacological treatments, more precise details on the balance of benefits and harms would have been needed before specific recommendations could be made.

In addition to the consensus-based recommendations described above, some specific recommendations are derived from more robust supporting evidence. For example, the recommendation for initiation of nonemergent antipsychotic treatment with a low dose of medication that is slowly titrated to the minimum effective dose (statement 8) is based on a substantial body of literature in geriatric pharmacology (Jacobson 2014; Lassiter et al. 2013; Mulsant and Pollock 2015; Wallace and Paauw 2015; Wooten 2012) as well as data suggesting that higher doses of antipsychotic medication are associated with a greater risk of harm in individuals with dementia (see section "Review of Supporting Research Evidence" in Appendix A). Statements 5, 8, 10, 14, and 15 are based on moderate-strength evidence in individuals with dementia that the benefits of antipsychotic medication are small. In addition, consistent evidence, predominantly from large observational studies, indicates that antipsychotic medications are associated with clinically significant adverse effects, including mortality, among individuals with dementia. The overall strength of evidence for these statements is graded as moderate on the basis of this balance of benefits and harms data and the fact that there were no studies that directly addressed all of the specific elements of each recommendation.

With respect to statement 12, harms data suggest a continued risk with ongoing treatment, and discontinuation studies show that medications can be tapered in many patients without symptoms recurring (see section "Review of Supporting Research Evidence" in Appendix A). The guideline writing group members were unanimous in recommending that an attempt at tapering and withdrawing the antipsychotic medication should be done for individuals being treated for psychosis or agitation in the context of dementia. One guideline writing group member (M.H.-L.) felt that an attempt at tapering is indicated for all individuals, where the patient's history of recurrence of symptoms during prior tapering attempts is an input to the tapering decision making along with other factors, as in statement 10. The strength of research evidence supporting statement 12 is rated as low because the precise timing of a tapering attempt was not studied in a randomized fashion and the recommendation to attempt a taper within 4 months was based on the timing of discontinuation in the available clinical trials and information from expert consensus (see sections "Review of Supporting Research Evidence" in Appendix A and "Expert Opinion Survey Data: Results" in Appendix B). Input from patients and their care partners, as well as comments from some geriatric psychiatrists, suggested that more flexible timing of a tapering attempt may be warranted. Some guideline writing group members also felt that a longer period of treatment may be justified in some patients before tapering is attempted because of the initial time needed to reach a clinically effective dose and the longer duration of psychosis in many patients as compared with the typical duration of agitated behaviors. It was also noted that for some patients, a medication taper could negatively affect quality of life or be dangerous for the patient or others. Some retrospective data also suggested that individuals with more severe symptoms may be at a greater risk of relapse with antipsychotic tapering, but the available research did not examine whether an a priori determination of such individuals would predict a high likelihood of symptom recurrence. Consequently, in the final guideline statement, the recommended attempt at tapering antipsychotics is accompanied by two additional recommendations. Statement 11 stresses the importance of patient, surrogate decision maker, and family input before a tapering attempt, as well as review of the clinical factors related to a tapering attempt, and statement 13 addresses the need for careful monitoring during tapering so that any recurrent symptoms can be addressed quickly.

For statement 14, the data on harms in observational and administrative database studies sometimes focused on specific medications and sometimes on the class of FGAs as compared with SGAs. Since haloperidol was the most commonly used agent among FGAs, it was difficult to determine whether other FGAs had a comparable risk of harms. For this reason, the group chose to recommend that haloperidol not be used as a first-line agent, rather than recommending against use of any FGA as a first-line agent.

For statement 15, there was an acknowledgement of potential benefits of a long-acting antipsychotic medication for adherence in some selected circumstances. Nevertheless, for the preponderance of patients, the potential harms of a long-acting formulation were viewed as greater than the potential benefits. However, there was recognition that under selected circumstances, this balance may shift. In particular, some individuals will have had a chronic psychotic disorder, such as schizophrenia, that preceded the onset of dementia, and clinical opinion suggests that these patients may have continuing benefits of long-acting antipsychotic medication.

## Limitations of the Evidence in Assessing Benefits and Harms

In assessing the balance between the benefits and harms of these recommendations, there are a number of factors to note. As our knowledge of dementia and its treatment evolve, there may be shifts in the balance of benefits and harms for these recommendations. At present, however, studies are either not available or not designed to give precise guidance on many of the clinical questions. One example is the lack of studies that examine benefits of assessment or discussion with patients, surrogate decision makers, families, and others. Another example is the small number of head-to-head trials comparing different pharmacological and nonpharmacological treatments for agitation or psychosis in dementia and an even fewer number of trials with parallel placebo or sham treatment arms. With nonpharmacological interventions, there can be significant variations in methodology from study to study, and multiple interventions can be administered together, confounding the interpretation of findings. Trials often fail to examine quality of life or other outcomes that patients and families view as most important. Studies also have not assessed the optimal time at which an attempted tapering of antipsychotic medication is indicated. There is insufficient evidence to determine whether individuals with more severe dementia, psychosis, or agitation will have a greater risk of relapse with antipsychotic discontinuation. In terms of monitoring, studies have not examined optimal timing of assessment during antipsychotic treatment or after an attempt at tapering antipsychotic treatment. The optimal frequency of laboratory and physical assessments to detect metabolic or other side effects of treatment also requires study in patients with dementia. It is also not clear whether laboratory data or other findings could predict which patients are at the highest risk of stroke or mortality or whether other interventions could reduce such risks.

Other aspects of research design may introduce variability into the findings and affect the ability to compare studies. A key issue is the way in which behavioral and psychological symptoms are defined and measured, with the definition and measurement of agitation being particularly problematic (Geda et al. 2013). Rating scales for behavioral and psychological symptoms define and measure agitation and aggressive behaviors in different ways and often mix measures of symptom frequency with measures of severity. New, shorter scales are also needed for routine clinical use. When studies have examined adverse effects of antipsychotic treatment in patients with specific subtypes of dementia, these diagnoses are generally based on clinical grounds, and this can introduce substantial variability as compared with diagnoses established through structured criteria, biomarker confirmation, or neuropathology (Beach et al. 2012). Studies with heterogeneous samples may fail to find a benefit or harm of a specific treatment, even if one is present for a more homogeneous subset of the patients.

As another source of variability, patients with dementia who are enrolled in clinical trials are not likely to be representative of the full range of individuals for whom clinical use of an antipsychotic medication might be considered. Significant physical illness (e.g., cardiopulmonary or renal impairments, cancer), use of certain medications (e.g., anticoagulants), or severe aggression requiring emergent intervention will typically exclude a subject from such research. Other psychiatric disorders, including substance use disorders, are also common exclusion criteria. It is not clear whether these typical exclusion criteria or other factors contribute to the apparent mismatch between clinicians' views of antipsychotic benefits and the limited benefits found in clinical trials. Nonetheless, these limitations of existing clinical trials make it hard to draw precise conclusions about the likely benefits of treatment for an individual patient.

In terms of harms data, typical administrative database studies are unable to show the temporal sequence between treatment and a specific outcome. Thus, an individual with dementia may fracture a hip, become delirious, and receive antipsychotic medication. An administrative database study would associate the hip fracture or a subsequent pulmonary embolus with antipsychotic medication even without a causal relationship. Alternatively, the presence of psychiatric symptoms such as agitation may result in both a greater risk of falls and an increased likelihood of receiving an antipsychotic medication (Lopez et al. 2013). In the future, prospective collection of harms data using registry reporting or electronic health record data analytics may help delineate the temporal sequence of antipsychotic use and adverse outcomes.

# Implementation

## Assessment of Behavioral/Psychological Symptoms of Dementia

In individuals with dementia who exhibit psychosis or agitation, initial assessment includes determining the type, frequency, severity, pattern, and timing of symptoms. Gathering this information typically requires multiple approaches, including interview and observation of the patient and review of relevant medical records. Flexibility is needed in adapting questions to the level of the patient's understanding and being sensitive to signs of frustration or cognitive overload (e.g., with formal cognitive testing) during the interview. The ability to answer questions can also be affected by language skills, educational achievement, or unrecognized impairments in hearing. Given that memory and other cognitive functions are impaired in individuals with dementia, it will probably not be feasible to obtain information on recent symptoms from direct questioning. On the other hand, a patient may minimize his or her difficulties or give a seemingly coherent response to a question about recent events despite having no actual recall. Thus, it is also important to obtain information from family members and other caregivers, including other treating clinicians and nursing facility or hospital staff.

Quantitative measures provide a structured replicable way to document the patient's baseline symptoms and determine which symptoms (if any) should be the target of intervention based on factors such as frequency of occurrence, magnitude, potential for associated harm to the patient or others, and associated distress to the patient. The exact frequency at which measures are warranted will depend on clinical circumstances. However, use of quantitative measures as treatment proceeds allows more precise tracking of whether nonpharmacological and pharmacological treatments are having their intended effect or whether a shift in the treatment plan is needed. Examples of available quantitative measures include the Neuropsychiatric Inventory Questionnaire (NPI-Q), which is Form B5 of the National Alzheimer's Coordinating Center Uniform Data Set (https://www.alz.washington.edu/NONMEMBER/UDS/DOCS/VER2/IVPforms/B5.pdf) (Kaufer et al. 2000) and Section E (Behavior) of the Minimum Data Set (MDS)—Version 3.0 of the Centers for Medicare & Medicaid Services Resident Assessment and Care Screening instrument (http://www.cms.gov/Medicare/Quality-Initiatives-Patient-Assessment-Instruments/NursingHomeQualityInits/index.html?redirect=/NursingHomeQualityInits/25_NHQIMDS30.asp), and the Brief Psychiatric Rating Scale (BPRS; Overall and Gorham 1988; Ventura et al. 1993), each of which incorporates measurement of agitation and psychosis. Alternatively, for individuals who are agitated but do not show evidence of psychosis, measures include the Cohen-Mansfield Agitation Inventory (CMAI; Cohen-Mansfield et al. 1989) or the four-item Modified Overt Aggression Scale (Kay et al. 1988). Although these measures and others have been used for reporting purposes as well as research (Gitlin et al. 2014), it remains unclear whether routine use of these scales in clinical practice improves overall outcomes. However, it is clear that each rating scale defines and measures psychosis, agitation, aggression, and other symptoms differently (Geda et al. 2013), making it preferable to use a consistent approach to quantitive measurement for a given patient. The extent of the assessment, including the use of quantitative measures, will be mediated by the urgency of the situation and by the time that is available for evaluation. Depending on the clinical circumstances, printed or electronic versions of quantitative scales may not be readily available or information may not be available to complete all scale items. If time constraints are present, the clinician may wish to focus on rating of relevant target symptoms (e.g., on a Likert scale). Another approach is for family or nursing facility staff to keep a log of target behaviors such as aggression and track the number of episodes that occur. In emergent circumstances, safety of the patient and others must take precedence; the initial assessment may need to be brief, with a more detailed assessment obtained once the acute clinical situation has been stabilized. If collateral sources of information are not immediately available, treatment may also need to proceed, with adjustments in the plan, if indicated, as additional knowledge is gained.

A careful assessment of the type, frequency, severity, pattern, and timing of symptoms will also serve as the foundation for determining potentially modifiable contributors to the patient's symptoms and identifying factors, such as the subtype of dementia (American Psychiatric Association 2013), that may influence choice of treatment. For example, pain is a common contributor to agitation (Bradford et al. 2012; Husebo et al. 2011; Kunik et al. 2010) but is not easily recognized because of sensory confusion and communication deficits (Pieper et al. 2013). Thus, priority should be given to identifying any source of pain and alleviating it through nonpharmacological and pharmacological approaches, as clinically indicated (American Geriatrics Society 2009). The pattern and timing of agitation may also suggest that the individual is becoming upset when he or she is hungry, fatigued, or cold or when there is a high amount of noise, clutter, or overstimulation in the environment. Vision or hearing deficits in combination with environmental factors can yield additive difficulties in an individual's ability to understand and cope with a situation. Interactions with caregivers may also have a temporal association with behavioral dyscontrol if the caregiver asks cognitively challenging questions, rushes the patient in carrying out tasks, or communicates his or her sense of anxiety or frustration, directly or indirectly. If the patient is being assisted with bathing, dressing, or other activities of daily living, rejection of care and agitation may be an outgrowth of many factors, including overstimulation, pain with particular movements, or the patient's sense of loss of control (Volicer et al. 2007). Attention to patient privacy needs is particularly important in assisting with activities of daily living. Constipation, incontinence, and other bowel or bladder issues can also prompt discomfort and distress. Other unmet needs may include, but are not limited to, relief from sensory deprivation, boredom, and loneliness (Cohen-Mansfield 2001).

Both precipitants and mitigating factors for agitation should be considered in the context of the patient's unique facets. These include the patient's likes and dislikes, lifestyle, hobbies, personality traits, intimacy and relationship patterns, spiritual and cultural beliefs, and past and current life circumstances. It can also be helpful to elicit information on prior aggressive behaviors (including associated legal problems), impulsivity, gambling, and problems with use of alcohol or other substances use. Using a person-centered approach calls for clinical staff to develop an understanding of the unique illness experience of the person and his or her care partners. This entails recognizing how individuals interpret the meaning of and navigate the difficult terrain associated with dementia and its symptoms. Input from the patient, his or her family members, and others (e.g., nursing facility or senior program staff) can give insights into patient preferences and the meaning of the behavior for the individual. It can also help in identifying approaches that have been helpful in managing agitation in the past and are therefore likely to be calming (Cohen-Mansfield et al. 2007). A person-centered approach also includes collecting information about previous traumatic experiences (e.g., childhood abuse, jail or prison experiences, domestic violence, combat experience, surviving the Holocaust, elder abuse) and possible triggers that may provoke inappropriate behaviors. Past life events, including traumas, are also relevant in terms of the resilience of the patient and his or her family as well as their previous approaches to coping with stress, loss, and decision making.

When interpreting the timing of symptom onset or worsening, clinicians should also consider changes in the patient's physical status such as a recent fall (e.g., associated with head injury or pain), onset of a medical condition (e.g., urinary tract infection, pneumonia), evidence of other psychiatric symptoms (e.g., depression, anxiety), or recent change in medications. Individuals may not take medications in prescribed doses at home; changes in adherence (e.g., due to forgetfulness, admission to or discharge from a hospital) may be associated with altered clinical response or toxicity. The Beers criteria provide a useful checklist of medications, such as benzodiazepines or anticholinergic agents, that may be particularly likely to cause side effects or toxicity in older individuals (American Geriatrics Society 2015 Beers Criteria Update Expert Panel 2015). In inpatient or nursing home facilities where medications have to be re-ordered at designated intervals, it is not uncommon for a medication to be inadvertently stopped. Given the sizable numbers of medications that many older adults are prescribed, it is also important to be mindful of the potential for drug-drug interactions or prescribing of multiple similar drugs. Toxicity with associated psychosis or agitation can develop with seemingly minor dose changes or medication additions. Furthermore, the reduced metabolism, altered distribution, and diminished clearance of medications in older individuals means that the time to achieve steady-state levels will be longer than in younger patients. With drugs that have a long half-life or a long-half-life active metabolite (e.g., aripiprazole, fluoxetine, clonazepam, diazepam), the full effects of a dose change may not be apparent for several weeks, and this fact should be considered before titration or tapering of such medications. The use of long-acting intramuscular depot formulations of medications can be particularly problematic in frail, older individuals because of the longer duration of effect and the inability to stop the medication if an adverse effect occurs.

Another important step is determining the exact nature of the symptom. For example, in an individual with visual or hearing impairments, sensory illusions and other perceptual distortions may occur; these must be distinguished from true hallucinations and delusions before decisions about interventions are made. Also, benzodiazepine use can be associated with disinhibition; restlessness or pacing may reflect medication-related akathisia. Whether a symptom such as psychosis or agitation will require intervention is dependent on how frequently the symptom occurs and whether it is associated with significant distress to the patient or potential harm to the patient or others. To determine the degree of distress and the severity of symptoms, the treating clinician will synthesize information from multiple sources, such as direct observations of behavior, verbalizations by the patient, and input from family members, others involved with the patient, and nursing facility staff (if relevant), to arrive at a clinical judgment.

With agitation and with psychotic symptoms, there can be considerable variability in manifestations and potential for risk. For example, a patient may respond very differently to a delusion that belongings have been stolen as compared with a delusion that his or her loved one has been kidnapped and replaced by an imposter. Irritability may presage verbal threats, pacing, or emotional outbursts, whereas in other individuals episodes of rage and severe physical aggression may develop without apparent warning. The potential risk to the patient or others of a particular set of symptoms may vary with the circumstances. Thus, the same behavior may be riskier in a patient residing at home with a frail spouse than in a well-staffed nursing facility.

## Development of a Comprehensive Treatment Plan

Given the complexities of addressing agitation and psychosis in individuals with dementia, it is important to develop and document a comprehensive plan of treatment that is an outgrowth of the assessment described above. Such a plan does not need to adhere to a defined development process (e.g., face-to-face multidisciplinary team meeting) or format (e.g., time-specified goals and objectives), but it should give an overview of the identified clinical and psychosocial issues along with a specific plan for further evaluation, ongoing monitoring, and nonpharmacological and pharmacological interventions, as indicated. Depending on the urgency of the initial clinical presentation, the availability of caregivers, and the time for assessment, the initial plan may need to be augmented over several visits and as more details of the history and treatment response are obtained.

If a symptom is rare, reassurance and redirection, with education of family and other caregivers, are likely to be sufficient, with other time-limited interventions used if needed. In some instances family members or other caregivers may find a symptom upsetting even when the patient is not distressed by it. For example, some patients experience visual or auditory hallucinations that are pleasant to them and not associated with anxiety or agitation. Other patients become verbally aggressive at times without physical aggression. Providing education and support to caregivers may aid them in coping with these symptoms (Brodaty and Arasaratnam 2012; Livingston et al. 2014).

If symptoms are more frequent and specific contributors to symptoms have been identified, these factors can be targeted for direct intervention. Common steps include treating underlying physical causes of psychosis or agitation and providing treatment for pain (Husebo et al. 2014). Mobility support, hearing aids, or eyeglasses should be used, when indicated. Some patients may respond positively to particular interventions (e.g., hand massage, pet therapy, music listening), whereas other patients may find the same nonpharmacological interventions upsetting or overwhelming, depending on their personal preferences and domains of cognitive impairment. Modifications to the environment can also be helpful such as optimizing lighting, reducing clutter, and removing items that the patient finds upsetting or that could be thrown or used as a weapon while agitated.

When individuals with dementia are residing in the community, behavioral symptoms such as agitation and psychosis can be extremely challenging for family and other caregivers to address (van der Lee et al. 2014). The associated impact on interpersonal relationships and increased caregiver burden can increase agitation and aggressive behaviors even further (Kunik et al. 2010). Psychosocial interventions that include individualized interpersonally based education and support for caregivers also appear to reduce the use of antipsychotic therapies in persons with dementia-related agitation (Richter et al. 2012). Education should increase knowledge, skills, and attitudes related to unmet needs, environmental regulation, and respect for individual preferences. One example of such an educational approach is the "Bathing without a Battle" training program (Gozalo et al. 2014). Clear communication of intended tasks, modification of caregiving strategies (e.g., bed baths vs. tub baths), or use of distraction to minimize the focus on caregiving can reduce combativeness and rejection of care (Galindo-Garre et al. 2015; Ishii et al. 2010). Additional strategies include use of therapeutic communication techniques (Cohen-Mansfield et al. 2007) and other approaches to challenging behaviors (Alzheimer's Association 2015; Glenner et al. 2005; Mace and Rabins 2011) that are appropriate for the person's level of impairment. Additional supports can be facilitated by treating clinicians and can be invaluable (Jensen et al. 2015; Tam-Tham et al. 2013), although their availability may depend on factors such as geographical accessibility of resources, financial constraints, insurance limitations, or other obligations of the caregiver (e.g., to work, to young children in the home).

Training in reflective practice can increase self-awareness and improve care by having staff or caregivers reflect on behavioral incidents in terms of what occurred, their own thoughts and feelings, their assessment of positives and negatives of the experience, their interpretations of possible contributors to the incident, and their conclusions about adaptations to make in the future. Frameworks for understanding agitated behavior (Cohen-Mansfield 2001) may suggest a focus on other factors such as unmet needs, positive rather than negative behaviors, reduced stimulation, or promotion of relaxation. In inpatient settings and nursing home facilities, attention to the culture of the treatment setting and availability of a sufficient number of staff will also be important if staff is to participate in education, develop new skills, and be able to apply them. When staff and caregivers learn to view and respond to agitation and aggression in a way that is less emotionally charged, it may also help offset compassion fatigue and burnout, which are often consequences of working with individuals with dementia.

In addition to nonpharmacological interventions, the treatment plan may include pharmacological interventions to address physical conditions or symptoms such as pain or constipation. Although outside the scope of this practice guideline, cholinesterase inhibitors or memantine for dementia, and medications for other psychiatric disorders such as depression or anxiety disorders, may also be part of the treatment plan. Monitoring of physiological parameters (e.g., weight, blood pressure), point-of-care testing (e.g., glucose fingersticks), or laboratory testing may be included when indicated. Other elements of the treatment plan will be unique to the individual and his or her past experiences, needs, desires, preferences, and values to provide comprehensive person-centered care that is aimed at alleviating distress, promoting comfort, and enhancing quality of life.

The plan of treatment should also be reassessed over time, with modifications made to address changes in the patient's cognitive status, symptom evolution, and treatment response. This may entail reassessing for contributing or mitigating factors as well as continuing effective behavioral interventions or environmental modifications, adding other approaches if symptoms are not well controlled, and discontinuing ineffective nonpharmacological approaches. Any prescribed medications should also be reviewed for their benefits and for evidence of adverse effects. For example, benzodiazepine use is common, despite minimal evidence of benefit (Defrancesco et al. 2015) and an association with an increased risk of falls (Woolcott et al. 2009), worsening of cognition (Defrancesco et al. 2015), and potentially increased mortality (Huybrechts et al. 2011).

## Assessment of Benefits and Risks of Antipsychotic Treatment for the Patient

Given the risks associated with antipsychotic medications, if nonemergent use of antipsychotic medication is being considered to address agitation or psychosis, it is important to review all aspects of the assessment and the treatment plan. The aims of such a review are to determine the frequency and severity of symptoms in a systematic fashion, identify consequences of agitation or psychosis (e.g., distress to the patient, danger to self or others), discover previously unrecognized contributors to agitation or psychosis, reassess the clinical response to nonpharmacological or pharmacological treatments, and decide whether different interventions might be indicated.

If agitation or psychosis results in significant negative consequences to the patient and to his or her quality of life, the potential for benefits of an antipsychotic medication should be weighed against the potential for harmful effects (see section "Potential Benefits and Harms" earlier in this guideline). This is particularly important given the modest benefits and demonstrated risks of antipsychotic treatment in clinical trials and in less rigorous observational and cohort studies. In emergent situations, when there is risk of harm to the patient or others, acute treatment may need to proceed to allow the immediate crisis to be stabilized. However, in other contexts, discussing potential benefits and harms with the patient's family or other surrogate decision makers and eliciting their concerns, values, and preferences are essential in helping them arrive at an informed decision about treatment that will be person-centered and focused on overall quality of life. Patients may also be able to appreciate these factors and offer input on their current and future treatment preferences depending on their level of cognitive impairment (O'Rourke et al. 2015). Open-ended questioning and discussion will likely be helpful in identifying potential benefits and side effects of treatment that are most important to the person living with dementia. For example, individuals may be particularly concerned about effects of the medication on their remaining capabilities in terms of cognition and communication. On the other hand, calming effects of medication may be viewed as particularly helpful if they ease distressing anxiety or suspiciousness or alleviate aggressive episodes, allowing individuals to remain safely in their homes. If medication calms the individual for even a few hours, it can facilitate attendance at an adult day program, giving them pleasure through program activities and granting a caregiver a few hours of respite. In all settings of care, such preferences of patients, family, and other caregivers should be respected, documented, and reviewed in ongoing discussions as part of the treatment planning process.

The subtype of dementia is another important factor to establish before the potential benefits and risks of antipsychotic treatment are considered (Chare et al. 2014; Mrak and Griffin 2007; Pressman and Miller 2014). For example, in individuals with Lewy body dementia and Parkinson's disease dementia, the risks of extrapyramidal side effects of antipsychotic medication and the potential for cognitive worsening will be significantly greater than in individuals with other types of dementia (Aarsland et al. 2005; Stinton et al. 2015) and in some instances have been reported to include irreversible cognitive decompensation or death. Although clozapine and quetiapine may be better tolerated than the other antipsychotic medications in these patients, the evidence for efficacy of these agents in treating psychosis is minimal (Stinton et al. 2015). Consequently, it may be better to avoid antipsychotic treatment for the visual hallucinations that are common among individuals with Lewy body dementia and for the psychotic symptoms with Parkinson's disease and dopamine agonist therapy. Individuals with frontotemporal lobar degeneration may also have a heightened sensitivity to antipsychotic medication (Pijnenburg et al. 2003). Even in individuals with a diagnosis of Alzheimer's disease, pathological evidence of Lewy body disease may be present (Mrak and Griffin 2007) and warrants review of diagnosis before antipsychotic medications are prescribed.

Other benefits and risks of treatment will relate to the individual characteristics and circumstances of the patient. For example, individuals with preexisting diabetes have an increased risk of hospitalization for hyperglycemia with antipsychotic initiation (Lipscombe et al. 2009), whereas those with preexisting problems with gait may be at an increased risk for falls if they develop extrapyramidal side effects. Lowering of blood pressure and development of orthostasis can also contribute to falls, particularly in combination with use of other medications or dehydration. Other co-occurring conditions such as cerebrovascular disease or cardiac disease may also influence the risk of side effects from antipsychotic medications. On the other hand, if agitation or psychosis is severe and distressing to the patient and can be reduced by judicious treatment with an antipsychotic, some individuals may experience an enhanced quality of life (Beerens et al. 2013) and be able to remain in the community for longer periods of time because of reductions in caregiver burden (Mohamed et al., 2012). When behavioral and psychological symptoms are associated with dangerous behaviors to the individual or to others, treatment with an antipsychotic medication may also be appropriate and can reduce risk.

## Dosing, Duration, and Monitoring of Antipsychotic Treatment

After a risk-benefit assessment and discussion with the family or other surrogate decision makers, if antipsychotic treatment is clinically indicated on a nonemergent basis, it is important to begin the medication at a low dose. Typical starting doses for frail or older patients will be one-third to one-half the starting dose used to treat psychosis in younger individuals or the smallest size of tablet that is available. Doses should be titrated gradually to the lowest dose associated with clinical response. Factors such as drug-drug interactions, medication half-life, and renal and hepatic function should be taken into consideration during titration of medications to avoid dose adjustments that are too rapid. Because of variations in the metabolism of antipsychotic medications and variations in the time needed to reach steady-state medication levels, it is not possible to predict the time needed to reach an adequate dose of medication for an individual patient. However, doses used in clinical trials in patients with dementia can serve as a guide to the typical dose of medication required with each agent.

As dose titration proceeds and at all points in the course of treatment with an antipsychotic, the clinician will want to assess the patient and obtain information from caregivers about response to treatment, possible medication side effects, and adherence. As described above, use of quantitative measures can be helpful in tracking longitudinal response. Poor adherence may be due to factors such as cost, difficulties with swallowing, resistance to taking medication, or intolerable side effects. If side effects are observed or reported, the nature, frequency, and severity of these side effects will determine whether the risks and benefits of treatment favor ongoing treatment, an attempt at tapering, or immediate discontinuation of the medication. Monitoring for tolerability is also important so that sedation, extrapyramidal effects, gait disturbance, cognitive impairing effects, and other side effects can be minimized. Specific recommendations about the timing of laboratory monitoring have not been developed for individuals with dementia who are being treated with antipsychotic medication; however, in individuals with schizophrenia, it has been suggested that an Abnormal Involuntary Movement Scale (AIMS) be done at least every 6 months in geriatric patients (American Psychiatric Association 2004). Monitoring blood pressure, weight, body mass index (BMI), waist circumference, fasting glucose, fasting lipid profile, and personal/family history have been suggested at baseline for individuals receiving antipsychotic medication, with additional personal/family history and waist circumference annually, blood pressure and fasting plasma glucose at 12 weeks and annually, lipid profile at 12 weeks and every 5 years, and weight with calculation of BMI monthly for 3 months, then quarterly (American Diabetes Association et al. 2004). Hemoglobin $A_{1C}$ monitoring may be substituted for a fasting glucose level (American Diabetes Association 2015).

If a partial response to antipsychotic treatment occurs, further dose titration may be indicated depending on whether side effects are present and on the relative balance of benefits and harms for the patient. When patients are being treated for psychotic symptoms, relief of distress or associated agitation may occur even though hallucinations or delusions persist. In such circumstances, further dose adjustments may not be necessary and would add to the potential for side effects. If there is no clinically significant response within 4 weeks of reaching a typical therapeutic dose of medication, the medication should be tapered and stopped to avoid potential harms of medication treatment without any offsetting benefit. If severe, dangerous, or significantly distressing symptoms persist, a trial of a different antipsychotic medication may be considered after reevaluation for contributing factors to the patient's symptoms, additional review of the risks and benefits of treatment, and discussion with the patient and surrogate decision maker, with input from family and other involved individuals.

Even when benefit is apparent, patients' symptoms and need for an antipsychotic medication may change. Consequently, in an effort to reduce the potential harms of treatment, an attempt should be made to taper the antipsychotic medication within 4 months of treatment initiation. However, earlier attempts at tapering the medication may also be warranted given the ongoing risk of harms with continued treatment.

In the same way that clinical and patient-specific circumstances will require clinical judgment in the decision to initiate treatment with an antipsychotic, the clinician will need to weigh multiple factors in a decision to attempt a taper of medication. Discussion with the patient, surrogate decision maker, family, or others involved with the patient is also important. The aim of such a discussion is to elicit their preferences and concerns as well as to review the initial goals, observed benefits, and side effects of antipsychotic treatment; potential risks of continued exposure to antipsychotics; and past experience with antipsychotic medication trials and tapering attempts. The duration of treatment before an attempt at tapering may depend on the chronicity of the symptom prior to treatment initiation and on the severity and degree of dangerousness of the target symptoms. If the initial reasons for antipsychotic medication treatment are unclear after information is obtained from treating health professionals, medical records, family members, or other sources of collateral information, an earlier attempt at tapering may be warranted. When symptoms have been long-standing or associated with significant physical risks, more caution will be needed in efforts at medication tapering. Similarly, if symptoms have recurred with previous tapering attempts, it may be appropriate to continue treatment without an attempt at tapering. In addition, this recommendation is not intended to apply to individuals with a preexisting psychotic disorder such as schizophrenia for whom ongoing antipsychotic treatment may be necessary. As with decisions about initiating antipsychotic treatment, it is essential to obtain input from patients, family, and other caregivers on an ongoing basis and review their preferences, values, and concerns about continued treatment or tapering in a person-centered fashion.

When a medication taper is attempted, close monitoring will be needed to note signs of recurrent symptoms, with monthly symptom assessments recommended during the taper and for at least 4 months after medication discontinuation. The nature of such assessment may vary and can include face-to-face assessments, telephone contact, or other approaches to following symptoms and behaviors. Again, it can be helpful to use quantitative measures or other structured approaches. If breakthrough symptoms are noted with tapering, this suggests that the benefit of the medication may outweigh the potential risks of continued treatment, that other contributing factors may need to be addressed, or that other nonpharmacological or pharmacological interventions may be indicated.

# Use of Specific Antipsychotic Medications, Depending on Clinical Context

If an antipsychotic medication is being initiated, a number of factors warrant consideration when a specific agent is being selected. For example, patients, surrogate decision makers, or family members may express a preference for a specific medication or note concerns about specific side effects (e.g., weight gain, diabetes, sedation, additional cognitive impairment). Such preferences should be considered in concert with the other factors noted below. Barriers to choice of specific medications are also common and typically involve regulatory stipulations, cost considerations, formulary coverage, or preauthorization requirements.

The potential side effects of specific medications are also important considerations. In studies using administrative databases that have examined a wide range of antipsychotics, the risk of mortality with an FGA in individuals with dementia was generally greater than the risk with an SGA. Head-to-head comparison data from randomized trials are limited, and the bulk of the available evidence on FGAs relates to haloperidol. Thus, because of the greater risk of harms with haloperidol treatment reported in clinical trials and cohort studies, this medication is not recommended as a first-line agent for nonemergent use in individuals with dementia. On the basis of the available data on harms, it may be preferable to avoid use of other FGAs as well. In emergent situations or in the context of delirium, use of haloperidol may still be appropriate, given its availability in an intravenous and short-acting intramuscular formulation and its relatively rapid onset of action relative to other parenteral antipsychotic medications. However, if longer-term treatment is indicated, a different agent should be chosen as a first-line medication.

Among the SGAs, the choice of a specific medication involves consideration of a number of factors. As described in the sections "Potential Benefits and Harms" earlier in this guideline and "Review of Supporting Research Evidence" in Appendix A, data from randomized placebo-controlled trials suggest efficacy for risperidone in treating psychosis and for risperidone, olanzapine, and aripiprazole in treating agitation. There was insufficient information from trials of quetiapine to determine whether it was efficacious in treating either agitation or psychosis, and it appeared to be no better than placebo in treating behavioral or psychological symptoms of dementia overall. In terms of potential risks, the pooled data from randomized trials indicate a greater risk of mortality with use of an SGA relative to placebo but do not show significant differences in mortality between placebo and individual antipsychotic medications. However, the total number of deaths in each study is small. When pooled placebo-controlled RCT data are considered along with data from larger observational cohort studies and research using administrative databases, the evidence suggests that there may be differences in risk between individual antipsychotic agents, but confidence intervals are overlapping and effects are dose dependent. In addition, the number of individuals who had received aripiprazole was very small relative to the number who had received risperidone or olanzapine. There is no information about the benefits or harms of asenapine, brexpiprazole, cariprazine, clozapine, iloperidone, lurasidone, paliperidone, or ziprasidone in individuals with dementia. The lack of head-to-head comparison data among antipsychotic medications on efficacy and on harms makes it difficult to designate a specific antipsychotic as being most appropriate to use as a first-line agent in treating agitation or psychosis in individuals with dementia.

As with all medication-related decisions, choice of a medication will also depend on factors such as the patient's prior responses to a specific agent; co-occurring medical conditions; the pharmacokinetic properties of the medication, such as absorption and half-life; and the potential for drug-drug interactions and additive side effects with other medications that the patient is already taking. Some antipsychotic medications have active metabolites of the parent drug that may be relevant in medication selection. For example, norquetiapine has significantly greater anticholinergic side effects than quetiapine; interactions of other medications with quetiapine's primary metabolic pathway (i.e., cytochrome P450 3A4) can also worsen anticholinergic effects. The side effect profile of a medication is another important factor in selecting a specific agent. In addition to the potential risk of serious adverse events such as mortality or stroke, commonly relevant side effects include sedation, hypotension, cardiac effects (including QTc interval prolongation), extrapyramidal effects, akathisia, falls, dysphagia with associated risk of aspiration pneumonia, effects on seizure threshold, and metabolic effects (including weight gain, diabetes, dyslipidemia, and metabolic syndrome). Anticholinergic effects of antipsychotic medications can worsen cognition or narrow angle glaucoma as well as contribute to urinary retention and constipation. The frequency of these adverse effects will vary depending on the antipsychotic medication that is chosen.

Features that individuals in the expert survey noted may influence their prescribing of specific medications include the long half-life, potential for drug-drug interactions, and partial agonist mechanism of action and rates of akathisia with aripiprazole; greater likelihood of extrapyramidal effects and hyperprolactinemia with risperidone; anticholinergic effects, sedation, metabolic effects, and weight gain with olanzapine; and QTc prolongation and changes in absorption with food for ziprasidone. For individuals with Lewy body dementia or Parkinson's disease dementia, quetiapine and clozapine were noted as the most appropriate medications because of the risk of worsened motor symptoms with the other antipsychotic agents.

The available formulations of the antipsychotic may also play a role in the medication selection process. For example, for patients who have difficulty swallowing pills, it would be preferable to choose a medication that is available as a rapidly dissolving tablet or oral concentrate formulation. If an intramuscular formulation of antipsychotic is indicated for short-term use in individuals who are unable to take oral medications or in emergent situations, care should be taken to use a short-acting parenteral preparation.

The long-acting injectable decanoate formulation of haloperidol and other long-acting injectable formulations of antipsychotic medications are likely to carry a greater risk of side effects in individuals with dementia. However, individuals with a chronic psychotic disorder, such as schizophrenia, may benefit from treatment with a long-acting injectable antipsychotic medication if they have a history of poor adherence and have tolerated oral formulations of medication. In other selected circumstances, a low dose of a long-acting injectable antipsychotic may aid adherence and minimize struggles over the taking of oral medications. Individuals with a preexisting chronic psychotic illness may also have adherence enhanced by administering long-acting medication. Nevertheless, if used, caution is needed to assure that oral medication is well tolerated before shifting to a long-acting injectable. Furthermore, care must still be taken in dosing of long-acting intramuscular formulations because of aging-related changes in medication pharmacokinetics, changes in body composition, and impairments in renal or hepatic function.

# Quality Measurement Considerations

This guideline includes 15 recommendations about the care of individuals with dementia who are exhibiting agitation or psychotic symptoms. Although the guideline focuses on the clinical indications (statement 5) and judicious use (statements 8 through 15) of antipsychotic medications to treat agitation or psychosis, other facets of care and clinical decision making are inextricably linked to decisions about pharmacological interventions. Thus, this guideline also incorporates recommendations about assessment of symptoms (statement 1), potentially modifiable contributors to symptoms (statement 2) and factors that may influence choices of treatment (statement 2), and approaches to monitoring of symptoms (statements 3 and 13). Other recommendations relate to having a documented plan of treatment (statement 4), reviewing response to nonpharmacological treatments (statement 6), and discussing the potential benefits and risks from antipsychotic medication (statement 7) or tapering of antipsychotic medication (statement 11) with the patient, if clinically feasible, and with the surrogate decision maker, with input from family and others involved with the patient.

## Existing Measures of Relevance to Antipsychotic Use in Individuals With Dementia

The recommendations of this guideline are consistent with several existing Choosing Wisely recommendations. For example, the American Psychiatric Association (2015a) advises, "Don't prescribe antipsychotic medications to patients for any indication without appropriate initial evaluation and appropriate ongoing monitoring" and "Don't routinely use antipsychotics as first choice to treat behavioral and psychological symptoms of dementia." The latter recommendation is echoed by the Choosing Wisely recommendation of the American Geriatrics Society (2015). In addition, two existing process measures relating to the use of antipsychotics in individuals with dementia have been endorsed by the National Quality Forum (NQF) (Pharmacy Quality Alliance 2014). For one of the measures (NQMC-9260), the denominator includes "patients 65 years and older with either a diagnosis of dementia and/or two or more prescription claims and greater than 60 days supply for a cholinesterase inhibitor or an N-methyl-D-aspartate receptor antagonist." The numerator is defined by "the number of patients in the denominator who had at least one prescription AND greater than 30 days supply for any antipsychotic medication during the measurement period and do not have a diagnosis for schizophrenia, bipolar disorder, Huntington's disease or Tourette's syndrome." The other measure (NQMC-9907) applies to long-stay nursing home residents with dementia who are age 18 years or older and examines the percentage of individuals who have been receiving an antipsychotic medication for 12 days or longer. Again, individuals with a diagnosis of schizophrenia, bipolar disorder, Huntington's disease, or Tourette's syndrome are excluded from the measure.

## Variability in Practice That May Be Addressed by Quality Measures

Available administrative data allow calculations of the rates of antipsychotic use in nursing homes (Partnership to Improve Dementia Care in Nursing Homes 2015) and other settings. Such data show significant regional and state-to-state variability; however, they have a number of confounds and do not provide details about the reasons these medications are being prescribed or the severity of symptoms exhibited by the patient. Thus, these data reflect antipsychotic use but, like the currently endorsed NQF measures, do not provide information about appropriate use of antipsychotic medications in individuals with dementia.

In terms of other recommendations, the typical practices of psychiatrists and other health professionals are unknown, but anecdotal observations suggest possible variability across healthcare settings and specialty practices. Such variability could indicate a need to strengthen clinician knowledge, improve training, or increase the time available to assess patients and document decision making. Variability could also indicate a need to address barriers to care such as geographic or socioeconomic differences in the availability of health professionals, skilled staff, specific medications, nonpharmacological interventions, or other care-related resources.

# Potential Options for Measure Development

Measures could be developed that focus on the assessment of behavioral and psychological symptoms in individuals with dementia, including the type, frequency, severity, pattern, and timing of symptoms (statement 1), potentially modifiable contributors to symptoms (statement 2), and factors that may influence choices of treatment (statement 2). The use of a quantitative measure (statement 3) would be difficult to implement as a quality measure because available rating scales are primarily designed for research. Less formal approaches to quantitative measurement would be better suited to typical clinical settings. Nevertheless, quantitative measures (statement 3) could be one option of several approaches for documenting symptom type, frequency, severity, pattern, and timing (statement 1). Typically, measures of assessment or screening should be matched to a measure that evaluates follow-up treatment and can therefore affect patient outcomes. Given the weak evidence for efficacy of nonpharmacological and pharmacological treatments for agitation and psychosis in dementia, pairing of a treatment-specific measure may not be appropriate. However, these measures could be paired with a measure relating to the presence of a documented treatment plan (statement 4).

Several recommendations (statements 5, 6, and 7) relate to the decision making that should precede consideration of nonemergency antipsychotic treatment in an individual with dementia. In particular, such treatment should be used only "when symptoms are severe, are dangerous, and/or cause significant distress to the patient" (statement 5), after "reviewing the clinical response to nonpharmacological interventions" (statement 6), and after assessing "the potential risks and benefits from antipsychotic medication" (statement 7). Statement 7 also recommends that "the potential risks and benefits from antipsychotic medication be assessed by the clinician and discussed with the patient (if clinically feasible) as well as with the patient's surrogate decision maker (if relevant) with input from family or others involved with the patient." This could be incorporated into the above measure as a process focused internal quality improvement measure, or a family/surrogate-reported satisfaction measure could be developed with patient input obtained, when clinically appropriate. For such measures, the measure denominator would focus on patients who received nonemergency treatment with an antipsychotic medication. Several other recommendations (statements 10 and 12) are related to attempts at tapering and discontinuing antipsychotic medications. Since many patients with dementia exhibit both agitation and psychosis and clinical responses can be subtle, it would be difficult to develop distinct measures to address each of these recommendations. However, a composite measure could be used to determine whether an attempt to taper the antipsychotic had occurred within 4 months of treatment initiation. Statement 11 also focuses on decision making and discussion with the patient, surrogate decision maker, and family, in this case related to tapering of antipsychotic medication in a patient who had experienced a positive response to treatment. The latter inclusion criteria would make it difficult to use this statement as a quality measure.

It may also be possible to develop a measure that assesses the use of haloperidol in individuals with dementia (statement 14). However, such a measure would require documenting whether or not the patient was experiencing delirium, whether or not the use of antipsychotic was on an emergency basis, and whether or not a different antipsychotic medication had been tried and stopped (e.g., due to side effects or lack of efficacy).

Other statements would be difficult or inappropriate to develop into quality measures because of the lack of a discrete and measurable numerator and denominator (statements 8, 9, and 13). Since long-acting injectable antipsychotic medications would be expected to constitute a small fraction of prescribed antipsychotic medications, the impact of a quality measure based on statement 15 is likely to be limited.

# Practical Barriers to Measure Development

For all of these recommendations, there are important practical barriers to the derivation and utility of quality measures. For example, to assess a clinician's performance of a clinical process, a measure must clearly define the applicable patient group (i.e., the denominator) and the process that is measured (i.e., the numerator). Furthermore, the clinician's performance of the process must be readily ascertained from chart review or administrative data. When quality measures relate to patient assessment, clinical judgment must be used to determine the factors that merit emphasis in the evaluation of an individual patient. Clinical judgment is also needed to determine the clinical response to nonpharmacological interventions, weigh the potential benefits and harms of antipsychotic treatment, and decide on the appropriate timing of attempts to taper antipsychotic medication.

Additional barriers relate to a lack of standardization in how findings are documented. Information in medical records may be lacking or incomplete; more often it does not fully align with the specific requirements of a particular performance measure. Many clinicians appropriately use free text prose to describe symptoms, response to treatment, discussions with family, plans of treatment, and other aspects of care and clinical decision making. Reviewing these free text records for measurement purposes would be impractical, and it would be inappropriate to hold clinicians accountable to such measures, without significant increases in electronic medical record use and advances in natural language processing. The presence or absence of scoring from a relevant measurement tool could be included as one of several approaches to fulfill a measure that relates to symptom assessment. Another approach could be to measure only for the presence or absence of text in relevant free text fields of an electronic medical record. This approach would allow for maximum flexibility in how clinicians document findings of their assessments; however, a liability of this approach is that it would have limited utility to address variability in how clinicians assess patients with dementia and document treatment planning and clinical decision making. Such an approach could also lead to documentation burden and overuse of standardized language that does not accurately reflect what has occurred in practice. On the other hand, if multiple discrete fields are used to capture information on a paper or electronic record form, oversimplification is a possible unintended consequence of measurement. For example, implementation of a measure relating to haloperidol use (statement 14) would minimally require that a clinician's medical record capture yes or no answers about current delirium, emergent need for treatment, and prior antipsychotic trials. Not all electronic medical records may do this without costly modifications, and even if they do, information may not be captured in an easily retrievable and reportable format. In addition, crucial clinical information might be lost through this type of documentation (e.g., information on responses or side effects from prior antipsychotic trials).

As a result of these practical barriers, it may be difficult to derive meaningful performance measures from these recommendations. Consequently, quality improvement activities including performance measures derived from these guidelines should yield improvements in quality of care to justify any clinician burden (e.g., documentation burden). Possible unintended consequences of any derived measures would also need to be addressed in testing of a fully specified measure.

# Additional Uses of Guideline Recommendations to Enhance Quality

In addition to the possible use of these guidelines to develop formal quality measures, these guideline statements can also be used to promote quality care in other ways. For example, quality of care might be improved through educational activities or through electronic clinical decision support. With appropriate controls for case-mix and comorbidities, organizations could examine the effects of the recommendations on overall outcomes (e.g., proportion of individuals with significant behavioral and psychological symptoms of dementia, proportion of individuals experiencing adverse effects of antipsychotic medication, rates of transition from community to nursing care settings). Quality improvement initiatives could then be developed to improve these outcomes.

# Guideline Development Process

This guideline was developed using a process intended to meet standards of the Institute of Medicine (2011). The process is fully described in a document available on the APA website: http://www.psychiatry.org/File%20Library/Psychiatrists/Practice/Clinical%20Practice%20Guidelines/Guideline-Development-Process.pdf. The development process included the following key elements.

## Management of Potential Conflicts of Interest

Members of the Systematic Review Group and Guideline Writing Group members were required to disclose all potential conflicts of interest before appointment, before and during guideline development, and on publication.

## Guideline Writing Group Composition

The Guideline Writing Group was initially composed of eight psychiatrists with general research and clinical expertise. To achieve a multidisciplinary group, some experts from other disciplines (i.e., nursing, neurology, and geriatrics) were added to the group. In addition, individuals nominated as experts on the topic were surveyed, as described under the section "Expert Opinion Survey Data: Results" in Appendix B. The Guideline Writing Group was diverse and balanced with respect to its members' expertise as well as other characteristics, such as geographical location and demographic background. Methodological expertise (i.e., with respect to appraisal of strength of research evidence) was provided by the Systematic Review Group. The Alzheimer's Association was involved in reviewing the draft and provided perspective from patients, families, and other care partners.

## Expert Opinion Data Collection

An expert opinion survey was fielded to 593 experts on the topic of the guideline. These experts were peer-nominated by current and past APA Council and work group members, chairs of academic departments of psychiatry, directors of psychiatry residency programs in the United States and Canada, leadership of other medical organizations, and the APA Assembly. Nominators were asked to identify two types of experts to serve on the panel: researchers and clinicians. "Research experts" were defined as individuals who have significant research activities, scholarly publications, or academic reputation in the treatment of Alzheimer's disease and other dementias, including the use of antipsychotic medications for the treatment of behavioral/psychological symptoms. "Clinical experts" were defined as individuals who have substantial clinical experience in the treatment of Alzheimer's disease and other dementias, including the use of antipsychotic medications for the treatment of behavioral/psychological symptoms. The experts were contacted via email to complete the survey online.

Survey questions were adapted from clinical questions developed by the AHRQ for its 2011 review on off-label use of antipsychotics (Maglione et al. 2011). The survey included questions to address appropriate antipsychotic use, duration of treatment, and clinical experience of using antipsychotics to treat agitation or psychosis in patients with dementia in given clinical circumstances.

Most of the experts, 66.2%, were nominated once, 14.7% were nominated twice, and the remainder were nominated up to 19 times. The composition of the portion of the experts who responded to the survey corresponds closely with that of the entire panel, within 0%–5% (i.e., in the number of times panel members were nominated and whether they were identified as clinical or research experts or both).

The response rate for the survey was 34.4% ($n=204$); 3.9% of the responses were partial, meaning that at least one question was completed. The experts who responded to the survey comprised approximately 61% clinical experts, 11% research experts, 24% experts in both categories, and 4% unspecified experts.

Quantitative data from the survey are shown in the section "Review of Supporting Research Evidence" in Appendix A. The survey also collected many free text comments, which were reviewed during development of the draft guideline. Key themes from qualitative data have been incorporated into the implementation section of the guideline.

# Systematic Review Methodology

This guideline is based on a systematic search of available research evidence. The search terms and limits used are available at http://psychiatryonline.org/pb-assets/books/Practice%20Guidelines/PG_Dementia_Search.pdf.

Initial searches of MEDLINE, PsycINFO, and Cochrane databases were conducted in February 2013 and included search terms for SGAs and for off-label indications for SGA use (including dementia), extending the search conducted for the AHRQ systematic review "Off-Label Use of Atypical Antipsychotics: An Update" (Maglione et al. 2011). These searches yielded 1,624 articles in MEDLINE, 657 articles in PsycINFO, and 1,457 articles in the Cochrane database. Two individuals (R.R. and L.J.F.) screened the 2,141 articles from the different searches when duplicate references were eliminated. Included articles were a clinical trial (including a controlled or randomized trial), observational study, meta-analysis, or systematic review that was clinically relevant to the off-label use of SGAs. The identified articles were subsequently restricted to the topic of dementia, and this yielded 12 articles (3 randomized trials, 9 observational studies).

Subsequent systematic searches were conducted in January 2015 and included terms for all antipsychotic medications and for all types of dementia, cognitive disorders, and cognitive impairment. Searches were limited to English language articles in adult humans and to clinical trials, observational studies, meta-analyses, and systematic reviews. All searches were done for the years from 1900 through 2014.These searches yielded 1,483 articles in MEDLINE, 470 articles in PsycINFO, and 335 articles in the Cochrane database. After duplicate articles and unpublished meeting abstracts were removed, two individuals (S-H.H. and L.F.) screened an additional 1,719 articles for relevance to the use of antipsychotic medications in individuals with dementia. Articles were included if they were randomized controlled trials that related to antipsychotic treatment of behavioral and psychological symptoms of dementia (BPSD). Because the AHRQ review (Maglione et al. 2011) only incorporated studies related to SGAs, we did not include randomized trials that only studied FGAs. We also excluded post-hoc analyses of pooled data and randomized trials that addressed acute use of intramuscular antipsychotic agents for the treatment of agitation. Observational studies, including administrative database studies, were included if they had a sample size of at least 500 individuals and addressed antipsychotic treatment of BPSD or harms of antipsychotic treatment in geriatric populations with or without dementia.

Results of this second search included all relevant articles that had been identified in the AHRQ review (Maglione et al. 2011) or in the initial search. Overall, 45 randomized controlled trials and 52 observational studies met the above criteria and were included in the guideline. An additional 4 studies appeared to meet these criteria upon screening the article title, but no abstracts were available and the full article could not be located. An additional 382 articles were related to dementia and antipsychotic treatment but did not meet the criteria noted above. Of these, 46 were meta-analyses or post-hoc analyses of pooled data and 13 were randomized controlled trials that only included an FGA. The remaining articles included 359 that were related to antipsychotic treatment but not dementia, 317 related to dementia but not antipsychotic treatment, and 560 that were unrelated to either dementia or antipsychotic treatment.

# Rating the Strength of Supporting Research Evidence

"Strength of supporting research evidence" describes the level of confidence that findings from scientific observation and testing of an effect of an intervention reflect the true effect. Confidence is enhanced by factors such as rigorous study design and minimal potential for study bias. Three ratings are used: high, moderate, and low.

Ratings are determined by the Systematic Review Group, after assessment of available clinical trials across four primary domains: risk of bias, consistency of findings across studies, directness of the effect on a specific health outcome, and precision of the estimate of effect. These domains and the method used to evaluate them are described above under "Systematic Review Methodology."

In accordance with the AHRQ's *Methods Guide for Effectiveness and Comparative Effectiveness Reviews* (Agency for Healthcare Research and Quality 2014), the ratings are defined as follows:

- **High** (denoted by the letter *A*) = High confidence that the evidence reflects the true effect. Further research is very unlikely to change our confidence in the estimate of effect.
- **Moderate** (denoted by the letter *B*) = Moderate confidence that the evidence reflects the true effect. Further research may change our confidence in the estimate of effect and may change the estimate.
- **Low** (denoted by the letter *C*) = Low confidence that the evidence reflects the true effect. Further research is likely to change our confidence in the estimate of effect and is likely to change the estimate.

# Rating the Strength of Recommendations

Each guideline statement is separately rated to indicate strength of recommendation and strength of supporting research evidence.

"Strength of recommendation" describes the level of confidence that potential benefits of an intervention outweigh potential harms. This level of confidence is informed by available evidence, which includes evidence from clinical trials as well as expert opinion and patient values and preferences. As described in the introduction to this guideline (see "Rating the Strength of Supporting Research Evidence"), the rating is a consensus judgment of the authors of the guideline and is endorsed by the APA Board of Trustees.

There are two possible ratings: recommendation or suggestion. These ratings correspond to ratings of "strong" or "weak" (also termed "conditional") as defined under the GRADE method for rating recommendations in clinical practice guidelines (described in publications such as Guyatt et al. 2008 and others available on the website of the GRADE Working Group at http://gradeworkinggroup.org/index.htm). "Recommendation" (denoted by the numeral 1 after the guideline statement) indicates confidence that the benefits of the intervention clearly outweigh harms. "Suggestion" (denoted by the numeral 2 after the guideline statement) indicates uncertainty (i.e., the balance of benefits and harms is difficult to judge or either the benefits or the harms are unclear).

When a negative statement is made, ratings of strength of recommendation should be understood as meaning the inverse of the above (e.g., "recommendation" indicates confidence that harms clearly outweigh benefits).

When there is insufficient information to support a recommendation or a suggestion, a statement may be made that further research about the intervention is needed.

The Guideline Writing Group determined ratings of strength of recommendation by a modified Delphi method using blind, iterative voting and discussion. In weighing potential benefits and harms, the group considered the strength of supporting research evidence, the results of the expert opinion survey, and their own clinical experiences and opinions. For recommendations, at least 9 of the 10 members of the group must have voted to "recommend" the intervention or assessment after four rounds of voting. On the basis of the discussion among the members of the group, adjustments to the wording of recommendations could be made between voting rounds. If this level of consensus was not achieved, the group could agree to make a "suggestion" rather than a recommendation. No suggestion or statement was made if three or more group members voted "no statement." Differences of opinion within the group about ratings of strength of recommendation, if any, are described in the section "Potential Benefits and Harms" earlier in this guideline.

# External Review

This guideline was made available for review on July 31, 2015 by stakeholders, including the APA membership, scientific and clinical experts, allied organizations (including patient advocacy organizations), and the public. A total of 44 individuals and 11 groups/organizations submitted comments on the guideline. The chair and co-chair of the Guideline Writing Group reviewed and addressed all comments received; substantive issues were reviewed by the Guideline Writing Group.

# Approval

The guideline was approved by the APA Board of Trustees on December 13, 2015.

# Glossary of Terms

**Adequate dose**  The dose of a medication at which therapeutic effects occurred when tested in clinical trials in a comparable population of subjects. This dose will differ for each medication and may need to be adjusted in an individual patient to address factors that would influence drug absorption, metabolism, elimination, or other pharmacokinetic properties.

**Adequate response**  A reduction in symptoms as a result of treatment that is associated with clinically significant benefit in functioning and/or quality of life. A reduction in symptoms of 50% or more is sometimes used as a threshold for adequacy of response.

**Agitation**  A state of excessive motor activity, verbal aggression, or physical aggression to oneself or others that is associated with observed or inferred evidence of emotional distress (definition adapted from Cummings et al. 2015).

**Antipsychotic medication**  One of a group of medications used in the treatment of psychosis. Some of the antipsychotic medications are also approved for use in other conditions such as mood disorders or Tourette's syndrome. The first-generation antipsychotic (FGA) medications, sometimes referred to as "typical" antipsychotic medications, were the initial medications to be discovered. The FGAs include, but are not limited to, chlorpromazine, droperidol, fluphenazine, haloperidol, loxapine, perphenazine, thiothixene, thioridazine, and trifluoperazine. The second-generation antipsychotic (SGA) medications, sometimes referred to as "atypical" antipsychotic medications, include, but are not limited, to aripiprazole, asenapine, brexpiprazole, cariprazine, clozapine, iloperidone, olanzapine, paliperidone, quetiapine, risperidone, and ziprasidone. Within each group of antipsychotic medications, there is significant variability in the pharmacological properties, presumed mechanisms, and side effect profiles of specific drugs.

**Assessment**  The process of obtaining information about a patient through any of a variety of methods, including face-to-face interview, review of medical records, physical examination (by the psychiatrist, another physician, or a medically trained clinician), diagnostic testing, or history taking from collateral sources.

**Behavioral and psychological symptoms of dementia**  Signs and symptoms of disturbed perception, thought content, mood, or behavior that occur in the context of dementia (Finkel et al. 1996). Behavioral and psychological symptoms of dementia (BPSD) are distinct from the cognitive impairments of dementia and include agitation and psychosis as well as apathy, depression, anxiety, irritability, disinhibition, sleep disturbances, wandering, and disruptive or socially inappropriate behaviors (Kales et al. 2015). This set of symptoms has also been referred to as noncognitive neuropsychiatric symptoms of dementia (Kales et al. 2014).

**Comprehensive treatment plan**  A plan of treatment that is developed as an outgrowth of the psychiatric evaluation and is modified as clinically indicated. A comprehensive treatment plan can include nonpharmacological and pharmacological interventions. It is individualized to the patient's clinical presentation, safety-related needs, concomitant medical conditions, personal background, relationships, life circumstances, and strengths and vulnerabilities. There is no prescribed format that a comprehensive treatment plan must follow. The breadth and depth of the initial treatment plan will depend on the amount of time and the extent of information that are available. The fully developed treatment plan will also vary in breadth and depth depending upon factors such as the needs of the patient and the setting in which care is occurring. Additions and modifications to the treatment plan are made as additional information accrues (e.g., from family, staff, medical records, and other collateral sources), and the patient's responses to clinical interventions are observed.

**Dementia**  A degenerative condition characterized by the development of multiple cognitive deficits that include memory impairment and at least one of the following cognitive disturbances: aphasia, apraxia, agnosia, or a disturbance in executive functioning. The cognitive deficits cannot occur exclusively during the course of a delirium; they must be sufficiently severe to cause impairment in occupational or social functioning, and must represent a decline from a previously higher level of functioning (American Psychiatric Association 2000). The definition of major neurocognitive disorder, as used in the *Diagnostic and Statistical Manual of Mental Disorders,* 5th Edition (DSM–5), is somewhat broader than the term *dementia,* in that individuals with substantial decline in a single domain can receive the diagnosis of neurocognitive disorder (American Psychiatric Association 2013).

**Nonpharmacological interventions**  Any of a wide variety of interventions other than medications. Nonpharmacological interventions include, but are not limited to, cognitive/emotion-oriented interventions (e.g., reminiscence therapy, validation therapy, simulated presence therapy, cognitive training and rehabilitation), sensory stimulation interventions (e.g., acupuncture, aromatherapy, light therapy, massage and touch therapy, music therapy, Snoezelen multisensory stimulation therapy), individualized behavioral reinforcement strategies, animal-assisted therapy, exercise, environmental modifications (e.g., reducing noise, decreasing clutter, removing access to sharp objects, establishing daily routines, providing orientation, improving lighting, increasing color contrasts), and caregiver support and education (Kales et al. 2015; O'Neil et al. 2011). Nonpharmacological interventions do not include restraint or seclusion.

**Quantitative measures**  Clinician- or patient-administered tests or scales that provide a numerical rating of features such as symptom severity, level of functioning, or quality of life and have been shown to be valid and reliable.

**Surrogate decision maker**  The individual who is designated to make decisions on behalf of the patient in circumstances where the patient lacks the capacity to do so. The specific designation of and terminology used to describe a surrogate decision maker will depend on state and federal law.

# References

Aarsland D, Perry R, Larsen JP, et al: Neuroleptic sensitivity in Parkinson's disease and parkinsonian dementias. J Clin Psychiatry 66(5):633–637, 2005 15889951
Adelman RD, Tmanova LL, Delgado D, et al: Caregiver burden: a clinical review. JAMA 311(10):1052–1060, 2014 24618967

*Note:* References to supporting research evidence are denoted by *. PubMed ID, where applicable, is included at the end of each reference.

Agency for Healthcare Research and Quality: Methods Guide for Effectiveness and Comparative Effectiveness Reviews. AHRQ Publication No. 10(14)-EHC063-EF. Rockville, MD, Agency for Healthcare Research and Quality. January 2014. Available at: http://www.ncbi.nlm.nih.gov/books/NBK47095/. Accessed February 8, 2016.

Alzheimer's Association: Caregivers for Alzheimer's and Dementia Face Special Challenges. Accessed October 1, 2015. Available at: http://www.alz.org/care/overview.asp.

American Diabetes Association: (2) Classification and diagnosis of diabetes. Diabetes Care 38(Suppl):S8–S16, 2015 25537714

American Diabetes Association; American Psychiatric Association; American Association of Clinical Endocrinologists; North American Association for the Study of Obesity: Consensus development conference on antipsychotic drugs and obesity and diabetes. Diabetes Care 27(2):596–601, 2004 14747245

American Geriatrics Society: Choosing Wisely. Available at: http://www.choosingwisely.org/clinician-lists/american-geriatrics-society-antipsychotics-for-dementia/. Accessed July 14, 2015.

American Geriatrics Society, Panel on Pharmacological Management of Persistent Pain in Older Persons: Pharmacological management of persistent pain in older persons. J Am Geriatr Soc 57(8):1331–1346, 2009 19573219

American Geriatrics Society 2015 Beers Criteria Update Expert Panel: American Geriatrics Society 2015 Updated Beers Criteria for Potentially Inappropriate Medication Use in Older Adults. J Am Geriatr Soc 63(11):2227–2246, 2015 26446832

American Psychiatric Association: Diagnostic and Statistical Manual of Mental Disorders, 4th Edition, Text Revision. Washington, DC, American Psychiatric Association, 2000

American Psychiatric Association: Practice guideline for the treatment of patients with schizophrenia 2nd Edition. Am J Psychiatry. 161(2 Suppl):1–56, 2004

American Psychiatric Association: Diagnostic and Statistical Manual of Mental Disorders, 5th Edition. Arlington, VA, American Psychiatric Publishing, 2013

American Psychiatric Association: Choosing wisely: five things patients and physicians should question. Available at: http://www.choosingwisely.org/societies/american-psychiatric-association/. Accessed July 14, 2015a.

American Psychiatric Association: Practice Guidelines for the Psychiatric Evaluation of Adults, 3rd Edition. Arlington, VA, American Psychiatric Association Publishing, 2015b

Andrews JC, Schünemann HJ, Oxman AD, et al: GRADE guidelines: 15. Going from evidence to recommendation-determinants of a recommendation's direction and strength. J Clin Epidemiol 66(7):726–735, 2013 23570745

Ayalon L, Gum AM, Feliciano L, Areán PA: Effectiveness of nonpharmacological interventions for the management of neuropsychiatric symptoms in patients with dementia: a systematic review. Arch Intern Med 166(20):2182–2188, 2006 17101935

Ballard CG, Thomas A, Fossey J, et al: A 3-month, randomized, placebo-controlled, neuroleptic discontinuation study in 100 people with dementia: the neuropsychiatric inventory median cutoff is a predictor of clinical outcome. J Clin Psychiatry 65(1):114–119, 2004 14744180*

Ballard C, Margallo-Lana M, Juszczak E, et al: Quetiapine and rivastigmine and cognitive decline in Alzheimer's disease: randomised double blind placebo controlled trial. BMJ 330(7496):874, 2005 15722369*

Ballard C, Lana MM, Theodoulou M, et al; Investigators DART AD: A randomised, blinded, placebo-controlled trial in dementia patients continuing or stopping neuroleptics (the DART-AD trial). PLoS Med 5(4):e76, 2008 18384230*

Ballard C, Hanney ML, Theodoulou M, et al; DART-AD investigators: The dementia antipsychotic withdrawal trial (DART-AD): long-term follow-up of a randomised placebo-controlled trial. Lancet Neurol 8(2):151–157, 2009 19138567*

Balshem H, Helfand M, Schünemann HJ, et al: GRADE guidelines: 3. Rating the quality of evidence. J Clin Epidemiol 64(4):401–406, 2011 21208779

Barak Y, Plopski I, Tadger S, Paleacu D: Escitalopram versus risperidone for the treatment of behavioral and psychotic symptoms associated with Alzheimer's disease: a randomized double-blind pilot study. Int Psychogeriatr 23(9):1515–1519, 2011 21492498*

Barnett MJ, Wehring H, Perry PJ: Comparison of risk of cerebrovascular events in an elderly VA population with dementia between antipsychotic and nonantipsychotic users. J Clin Psychopharmacol 27(6):595–601, 2007 18004126*

Beach TG, Monsell SE, Phillips LE, Kukull W: Accuracy of the clinical diagnosis of Alzheimer disease at National Institute on Aging Alzheimer Disease Centers, 2005-2010. J Neuropathol Exp Neurol 71(4):266–273, 2012 22437338

Beerens HC, Zwakhalen SM, Verbeek H, et al: Factors associated with quality of life of people with dementia in long-term care facilities: a systematic review. Int J Nurs Stud 50(9):1259–1270, 2013 23465959

Bradford A, Shrestha S, Snow AL, et al: Managing pain to prevent aggression in people with dementia: a non-pharmacologic intervention. Am J Alzheimers Dis Other Demen 27(1):41–47, 2012 22467413

Brasure M, Jutkowitz E, Fuchs E, et al: Nonpharmacologic Interventions for Agitation and Aggression in Dementia. Comparative Effectiveness Review No 177. (Prepared by the Minnesota Evidence-based Practice Center under Contract No. 290-2012-00016-I.) AHRQ Publ No 16-EHC019-EF. Rockville, MD, Agency for Healthcare Research and Quality, March 2016. Available at: https://www.effectivehealthcare.ahrq.gov/search-for-guides-reviews-and-reports/?pageaction=displayproduct&productID=2198. Accessed March 22, 2016.

Breder C, Swanink R, Marcus R, et al: Dose-ranging study of aripiprazole in patients with dementia of Alzheimer's disease. Neurobiol Aging 25(suppl):S190, 2004*

Brito JP, Domecq JP, Murad MH, et al: The Endocrine Society guidelines: when the confidence cart goes before the evidence horse. J Clin Endocrinol Metab 98(8):3246–3252, 2013 23783104

Brodaty H, Ames D, Snowdon J, et al: A randomized placebo-controlled trial of risperidone for the treatment of aggression, agitation, and psychosis of dementia. J Clin Psychiatry 64(2):134–143, 2003 12633121*

Brodaty H, Ames D, Snowdon J, et al: Risperidone for psychosis of Alzheimer's disease and mixed dementia: results of a double-blind, placebo-controlled trial. Int J Geriatr Psychiatry 20(12):1153–1157, 2005 16315159*

Brodaty H, Arasaratnam C: Meta-analysis of nonpharmacological interventions for neuropsychiatric symptoms of dementia. Am J Psychiatry 169(9):946–953, 2012 22952073

Brookmeyer R, Johnson E, Ziegler-Graham K, Arrighi HM: Forecasting the global burden of Alzheimer's disease. Alzheimers Dement 3(3):186–191, 2007 19595937

Chan MC, Chong CS, Wu AY, et al: Antipsychotics and risk of cerebrovascular events in treatment of behavioural and psychological symptoms of dementia in Hong Kong: a hospital-based, retrospective, cohort study. Int J Geriatr Psychiatry 25(4):362–370, 2010 19650162*

Chan TC, Luk JK, Shea YF, et al: Continuous use of antipsychotics and its association with mortality and hospitalization in institutionalized Chinese older adults: an 18-month prospective cohort study. Int Psychogeriatr 23(10):1640–1648, 2011 21902863*

Chan WC, Lam LC, Choy CN, et al: A double-blind randomised comparison of risperidone and haloperidol in the treatment of behavioural and psychological symptoms in Chinese dementia patients. Int J Geriatr Psychiatry 16(12):1156–1162, 2001 11748775*

Chare L, Hodges JR, Leyton CE, et al: New criteria for frontotemporal dementia syndromes: clinical and pathological diagnostic implications. J Neurol Neurosurg Psychiatry 85(8):865–870, 2014 24421286

Chatterjee S, Chen H, Johnson ML, Aparasu RR: Comparative risk of cerebrovascular adverse events in community-dwelling older adults using risperidone, olanzapine and quetiapine: a multiple propensity score-adjusted retrospective cohort study. Drugs Aging 29(10):807–817, 2012 23018582*

Cohen-Mansfield J: Nonpharmacologic interventions for inappropriate behaviors in dementia: a review, summary, and critique. Am J Geriatr Psychiatry 9(4):361–381, 2001 11739063

Cohen-Mansfield J, Marx MS, Rosenthal AS: A description of agitation in a nursing home. J Gerontol 44(3):M77–M84, 1989 2715584

Cohen-Mansfield J, Libin A, Marx MS: Nonpharmacological treatment of agitation: a controlled trial of systematic individualized intervention. J Gerontol A Biol Sci Med Sci 62(8):908–916, 2007 17702884

Corbett A, Burns A, Ballard C: Don't use antipsychotics routinely to treat agitation and aggression in people with dementia. BMJ 349:g6420, 2014 25368388

Council of Medical Specialty Societies (CMSS): Principles for the Development of Specialty Society Clinical Guidelines. Chicago, IL, Council of Medical Specialty Societies, 2012

Culo S, Mulsant BH, Rosen J, et al: Treating neuropsychiatric symptoms in dementia with Lewy bodies: a randomized controlled-trial. Alzheimer Dis Assoc Disord 24(4):360–364, 2010 20625270*

Cummings J, Mintzer J, Brodaty H, et al; International Psychogeriatric Association: Agitation in cognitive disorders: International Psychogeriatric Association provisional consensus clinical and research definition. Int Psychogeriatr 27(1):7–17, 2015 25311499

Dauphinot V, Delphin-Combe F, Mouchoux C, et al: Risk factors of caregiver burden among patients with Alzheimer's disease or related disorders: a cross-sectional study. J Alzheimers Dis 44(3):907–916, 2015 25374109

Deberdt WG, Dysken MW, Rappaport SA, et al: Comparison of olanzapine and risperidone in the treatment of psychosis and associated behavioral disturbances in patients with dementia. Am J Geriatr Psychiatry 13(8):722–730, 2005 16085789*

Declercq T, Petrovic M, Azermai M, et al: Withdrawal versus continuation of chronic antipsychotic drugs for behavioural and psychological symptoms in older people with dementia. Cochrane Database Syst Rev 3:CD007726, 2013 23543555

De Deyn PP, Rabheru K, Rasmussen A, et al: A randomized trial of risperidone, placebo, and haloperidol for behavioral symptoms of dementia. Neurology 53(5):946–955, 1999 10496251*

De Deyn PP, Carrasco MM, Deberdt W, et al: Olanzapine versus placebo in the treatment of psychosis with or without associated behavioral disturbances in patients with Alzheimer's disease. Int J Geriatr Psychiatry 19(2):115–126, 2004 14758577*

De Deyn PP, Jeste DV, Swanink R, et al: Aripiprazole for the treatment of psychosis in patients with Alzheimer's disease: a randomized, placebo-controlled study. J Clin Psychopharmacol 25(5):463–467, 2005 16160622*

De Deyn PP, Eriksson H, Svensson H; Study 115 investigators: Tolerability of extended-release quetiapine fumarate compared with immediate-release quetiapine fumarate in older patients with Alzheimer's disease with symptoms of psychosis and/or agitation: a randomised, double-blind, parallel-group study. Int J Geriatr Psychiatry 27(3):296–304, 2012 21538537*

Defrancesco M, Marksteiner J, Fleischhacker WW, Blasko I: Use of benzodiazepines in Alzheimer's disease: a systematic review of literature. Int J Neuropsychopharmacol 18(10):pyv055, 2015 25991652

Devanand DP, Pelton GH, Cunqueiro K, et al: A 6-month, randomized, double-blind, placebo-controlled pilot discontinuation trial following response to haloperidol treatment of psychosis and agitation in Alzheimer's disease. Int J Geriatr Psychiatry 26(9):937–943, 2011 21845596*

Devanand DP, Mintzer J, Schultz SK, et al: Relapse risk after discontinuation of risperidone in Alzheimer's disease. N Engl J Med 367(16):1497–1507, 2012 23075176*

de Vugt ME, Stevens F, Aalten P, et al: A prospective study of the effects of behavioral symptoms on the institutionalization of patients with dementia. Int Psychogeriatr 17(4):577–589, 2005 16185379

Djulbegovic B, Trikalinos TA, Roback J, et al: Impact of quality of evidence on the strength of recommendations: an empirical study. BMC Health Serv Res 9:120, 2009 19622148

Dutcher SK, Rattinger GB, Langenberg P, et al: Effect of medications on physical function and cognition in nursing home residents with dementia. J Am Geriatr Soc 62(6):1046–1055, 2014 24823451*

Ferri CP, Prince M, Brayne C, et al; Alzheimer's Disease International: Global prevalence of dementia: a Delphi consensus study. Lancet 366(9503):2112–2117, 2005 16360788

Finkel SI, Costa e Silva J, Cohen G, et al: Behavioral and psychological signs and symptoms of dementia: a consensus statement on current knowledge and implications for research and treatment. Int Psychogeriatr 8 (suppl 3):497–500, 1996 9154615

Finkel S, Kozma C, Long S, et al: Risperidone treatment in elderly patients with dementia: relative risk of cerebrovascular events versus other antipsychotics. Int Psychogeriatr 17(4):617–629, 2005 16202186*

Fontaine CS, Hynan LS, Koch K, et al: A double-blind comparison of olanzapine versus risperidone in the acute treatment of dementia-related behavioral disturbances in extended care facilities. J Clin Psychiatry 64(6):726–730, 2003 12823090*

Freund-Levi Y, Bloniecki V, Auestad B, et al: Galantamine versus risperidone for agitation in people with dementia: a randomized, twelve-week, single-center study. Dement Geriatr Cogn Disord 38(3-4):234–244, 2014a 24969380*

Freund-Levi Y, Jedenius E, Tysen-Bäckström AC, et al: Galantamine versus risperidone treatment of neuropsychiatric symptoms in patients with probable dementia: an open randomized trial. Am J Geriatr Psychiatry 22(4):341–348, 2014b 24035407*

Galindo-Garre F, Volicer L, van der Steen JT: Factors related to rejection of care and behaviors directed towards others: a longitudinal study in nursing home residents with dementia. Dement Geriatr Cogn Dis Extra 5(1):123–134, 2015 25999979

Gardette V, Lapeyre-Mestre M, Coley N, et al: Antipsychotic use and mortality risk in community-dwelling Alzheimer's disease patients: evidence for a role of dementia severity. Curr Alzheimer Res 9(9):1106–1116, 2012 22950915*

Gareri P, Cotroneo A, Lacava R, et al: Comparison of the efficacy of new and conventional antipsychotic drugs in the treatment of behavioral and psychological symptoms of dementia (BPSD). Arch Gerontol Geriatr Suppl 9:207–215, 2004 15207416*

Geda YE, Schneider LS, Gitlin LN, et al; Neuropsychiatric Syndromes Professional Interest Area of ISTAART: Neuropsychiatric symptoms in Alzheimer's disease: past progress and anticipation of the future. Alzheimers Dement 9(5):602–608, 2013 23562430

Gerhard T, Huybrechts K, Olfson M, et al: Comparative mortality risks of antipsychotic medications in community-dwelling older adults. Br J Psychiatry 205(1):44–51, 2014 23929443*

Gill SS, Rochon PA, Herrmann N, et al: Atypical antipsychotic drugs and risk of ischaemic stroke: population based retrospective cohort study. BMJ 330(7489):445, 2005 15668211*

Gill SS, Bronskill SE, Normand SL, et al: Antipsychotic drug use and mortality in older adults with dementia. Ann Intern Med 146(11):775–786, 2007 17548409*

Gisev N, Hartikainen S, Chen TF, et al: Effect of comorbidity on the risk of death associated with antipsychotic use among community-dwelling older adults. Int Psychogeriatr 24(7):1058–1064, 2012 22364618*

Gitlin LN, Hodgson N, Jutkowitz E, Pizzi L: The cost-effectiveness of a nonpharmacologic intervention for individuals with dementia and family caregivers: the tailored activity program. Am J Geriatr Psychiatry 18(6):510–519, 2010 20847903

Gitlin LN, Marx KA, Stanley IH, et al: Assessing neuropsychiatric symptoms in people with dementia: a systematic review of measures. Int Psychogeriatr 26(11):1805–1848, 2014 25096416

Glenner JA, Stehman JM, Davagnino J, et al: When your loved one has dementia: A simple guide for caregivers. Baltimore: Johns Hopkins University Press, 2005

Gozalo P, Prakash S, Qato DM, et al: Effect of the bathing without a battle training intervention on bathing-associated physical and verbal outcomes in nursing home residents with dementia: a randomized crossover diffusion study. J Am Geriatr Soc 62(5):797–804, 2014 24697702

Guyatt G, Gutterman D, Baumann MH, et al: Grading strength of recommendations and quality of evidence in clinical guidelines: report from an American College of Chest Physicians task force. Chest 129(1):174–181, 2006 16424429

Guyatt G, Eikelboom JW, Akl EA, et al: A guide to GRADE guidelines for the readers of JTH. J Thromb Haemost 11(8):1603–1608, 2013 23773710

Guyatt GH, Oxman AD, Kunz R, et al; GRADE Working Group: Going from evidence to recommendations. BMJ 336(7652):1049–1051, 2008 18467413

Hazlehurst JM, Armstrong MJ, Sherlock M, et al: A comparative quality assessment of evidence-based clinical guidelines in endocrinology. Clin Endocrinol (Oxf) 78(2):183–190, 2013 22624723

Hebert LE, Weuve J, Scherr PA, Evans DA: Alzheimer disease in the United States (2010-2050) estimated using the 2010 census. Neurology 80(19):1778–1783, 2013 23390181

Herrmann N, Mamdani M, Lanctôt KL: Atypical antipsychotics and risk of cerebrovascular accidents. Am J Psychiatry 161(6):1113–1115, 2004 15169702*

Hollis J, Grayson D, Forrester L, et al: Antipsychotic medication dispensing and risk of death in veterans and war widows 65 years and older. Am J Geriatr Psychiatry 15(11):932–941, 2007 17974865*

Holmes C, Wilkinson D, Dean C, et al: Risperidone and rivastigmine and agitated behaviour in severe Alzheimer's disease: a randomised double blind placebo controlled study. Int J Geriatr Psychiatry 22(4):380–381, 2007 17380475*

Husebo BS, Ballard C, Aarsland D: Pain treatment of agitation in patients with dementia: a systematic review. Int J Geriatr Psychiatry 26(10):1012–1018, 2011 21308784

Husebo BS, Ballard C, Cohen-Mansfield J, et al: The response of agitated behavior to pain management in persons with dementia. Am J Geriatr Psychiatry 22(7):708–717, 2014 23611363

Huybrechts KF, Rothman KJ, Silliman RA, et al: Risk of death and hospital admission for major medical events after initiation of psychotropic medications in older adults admitted to nursing homes. CMAJ 183(7):E411–E419, 2011 21444611*

Huybrechts KF, Gerhard T, Crystal S, et al: Differential risk of death in older residents in nursing homes prescribed specific antipsychotic drugs: population based cohort study. BMJ 344:e977, 2012 22362541*

Imfeld P, Bodmer M, Schuerch M, et al: Risk of incident stroke in patients with Alzheimer disease or vascular dementia. Neurology 81(10):910–919, 2013 23902701*

Institute of Medicine: Clinical Practice Guidelines We Can Trust. Washington, DC, National Academies Press, 2011

Ishii S, Streim JE, Saliba D: Potentially reversible resident factors associated with rejection of care behaviors. J Am Geriatr Soc 58(9):1693–1700, 2010 20863329

Jacobson SA: Clinical Manual of Geriatric Psychopharmacology, 2nd Edition. Arlington, VA, American Psychiatric Publishing, 2014

Jadad AR, Moore RA, Carroll D, et al: Assessing the quality of reports of randomized clinical trials: is blinding necessary? Control Clin Trials 17(1):1–12, 1996 8721797

Jalbert JJ, Eaton CB, Miller SC, Lapane KL: Antipsychotic use and the risk of hip fracture among older adults afflicted with dementia. J Am Med Dir Assoc 11(2):120–127, 2010 20142067*

Jalbert JJ, Daiello LA, Eaton CB, et al: Antipsychotic use and the risk of diabetes in nursing home residents with dementia. Am J Geriatr Pharmacother 9(3):153–163, 2011 21596626*

Jensen M, Agbata IN, Canavan M, McCarthy G: Effectiveness of educational interventions for informal caregivers of individuals with dementia residing in the community: systematic review and meta-analysis of randomised controlled trials. Int J Geriatr Psychiatry 30(2):130–143, 2015 25354132

Kales HC, Valenstein M, Kim HM, et al: Mortality risk in patients with dementia treated with antipsychotics versus other psychiatric medications. Am J Psychiatry 164(10):1568–1576, quiz 1623, 2007 17898349*

Kales HC, Kim HM, Zivin K, et al: Risk of mortality among individual antipsychotics in patients with dementia. Am J Psychiatry 169(1):71–79, 2012 22193526*

Kales HC, Gitlin LN, Lyketsos CG; Detroit Expert Panel on Assessment and Management of Neuropsychiatric Symptoms of Dementia: Management of neuropsychiatric symptoms of dementia in clinical settings: recommendations from a multidisciplinary expert panel. J Am Geriatr Soc 62(4):762–769, 2014 24635665

Kales HC, Gitlin LN, Lyketsos CG: Assessment and management of behavioral and psychological symptoms of dementia. BMJ 350:h369, 2015 25731881

Katz IR, Jeste DV, Mintzer JE, et al; Risperidone Study Group: Comparison of risperidone and placebo for psychosis and behavioral disturbances associated with dementia: a randomized, double-blind trial. J Clin Psychiatry 60(2):107–115, 1999 10084637*

Kaufer DI, Cummings JL, Ketchel P, et al: Validation of the NPI-Q, a brief clinical form of the Neuropsychiatric Inventory. J Neuropsychiatry Clin Neurosci 12(2):233–239, 2000 11001602*

Kay SR, Wolkenfeld F, Murrill LM: Profiles of aggression among psychiatric patients. I. Nature and prevalence. J Nerv Ment Dis 176(9):539–546, 1988 3418327

Kleijer BC, van Marum RJ, Egberts AC, et al: Risk of cerebrovascular events in elderly users of antipsychotics. J Psychopharmacol 23(8):909–914, 2009 18635700*

Knol W, van Marum RJ, Jansen PA, et al: Antipsychotic drug use and risk of pneumonia in elderly people. J Am Geriatr Soc 56(4):661–666, 2008 18266664*

Kong EH, Evans LK, Guevara JP: Nonpharmacological intervention for agitation in dementia: a systematic review and meta-analysis. Aging Ment Health 13(4):512–520, 2009 19629775

Kunik ME, Snow AL, Davila JA, et al: Causes of aggressive behavior in patients with dementia. J Clin Psychiatry 71(9):1145–1152, 2010 20361896

Langballe EM, Engdahl B, Nordeng H, et al: Short- and long-term mortality risk associated with the use of antipsychotics among 26,940 dementia outpatients: a population-based study. Am J Geriatr Psychiatry 22(4):321–331, 2014 24016844*

Laredo L, Vargas E, Blasco AJ, et al: Risk of cerebrovascular accident associated with use of antipsychotics: population-based case-control study. J Am Geriatr Soc 59(7):1182–1187, 2011 21718267*

Lassiter J, Bennett WM, Olyaei AJ: Drug dosing in elderly patients with chronic kidney disease. Clin Geriatr Med 29(3):657–705, 2013 23849014

Lee PE, Sykora K, Gill SS, et al: Antipsychotic medications and drug-induced movement disorders other than parkinsonism: a population-based cohort study in older adults. J Am Geriatr Soc 53:1374–1379, 2005 16078964*

Liperoti R, Gambassi G, Lapane KL, et al: Cerebrovascular events among elderly nursing home patients treated with conventional or atypical antipsychotics. J Clin Psychiatry 66:1090–1096, 2005 16187764*

Liperoti R, Onder G, Landi F, et al: All-cause mortality associated with atypical and conventional antipsychotics among nursing home residents with dementia: a retrospective cohort study. J Clin Psychiatry 70(10):1340–1347, 2009 19906339*

Lipkovich I, Ahl J, Nichols R, et al: Weight changes during treatment with olanzapine in older adult patients with dementia and behavioral disturbances. J Geriatr Psychiatry Neurol 20(2):107–114, 2007 17548781*

Lipscombe LL, Lévesque L, Gruneir A, et al: Antipsychotic drugs and hyperglycemia in older patients with diabetes. Arch Intern Med 169(14):1282–1289, 2009 19636029

Lipscombe LL, Lévesque LE, Gruneir A, et al: Antipsychotic drugs and the risk of hyperglycemia in older adults without diabetes: a population-based observational study. Am J Geriatr Psychiatry 19(12):1026–1033, 2011 22123274*

Liu ME, Tsai SJ, Chang WC, et al: Population-based 5-year follow-up study in Taiwan of dementia and risk of stroke. PLoS ONE 8(4):e61771, 2013 23626726*

Livingston G, Kelly L, Lewis-Holmes E, et al: Non-pharmacological interventions for agitation in dementia: systematic review of randomised controlled trials. Br J Psychiatry 205(6):436–442, 2014 25452601

Lopez OL, Becker JT, Chang Y-F, et al: The long-term effects of conventional and atypical antipsychotics in patients with probable Alzheimer's disease. Am J Psychiatry 170(9):1051–1058, 2013 23896958*

Lyketsos CG, Steinberg M, Tschanz JT, et al: Mental and behavioral disturbances in dementia: findings from the Cache County Study on Memory in Aging. Am J Psychiatry 157(5):708–714, 2000 10784462

Lyketsos CG, Lopez O, Jones B, et al: Prevalence of neuropsychiatric symptoms in dementia and mild cognitive impairment: results from the cardiovascular health study. JAMA 288(12):1475–1483, 2002 12243634

Mace NL, Rabins PV: The 36-hour day: A family guide to caring for people who have Alzheimer disease, related dementias, and memory loss. 5th ed. Baltimore: Johns Hopkins University Press, 2011

Maglione M, Ruelaz Maher A, Hu J, et al: Off-Label Use of Atypical Antipsychotics: An Update. Comparative Effectiveness Review No. 43. (Prepared by the Southern California Evidence-based Practice Center under Contract No. HHSA290-2007-10062-1.) Rockville, MD, Agency for Healthcare Research and Quality, September 2011. Available at: www.effectivehealthcare.ahrq.gov/reports/final.cfm.*

Marras C, Herrmann N, Anderson GM, et al: Atypical antipsychotic use and parkinsonism in dementia: effects of drug, dose, and sex. Am J Geriatr Pharmacother 10(6):381–389, 2012 23217531*

Maust DT, Kim HM, Seyfried LS, et al: Antipsychotics, other psychotropics, and the risk of death in patients with dementia: number needed to harm. JAMA Psychiatry 72(5):438–445, 2015 25786075

Micca JL, Hoffmann VP, Lipkovich I, et al: Retrospective analysis of diabetes risk in elderly patients with dementia in olanzapine clinical trials. Am J Geriatr Psychiatry 14(1):62–70, 2006 16407583*

Miller EA, Rosenheck RA, Schneider LS: Caregiver burden, health utilities, and institutional service use in Alzheimer's disease. Int J Geriatr Psychiatry 27(4):382–393, 2012 21560160

Mintzer J, Greenspan A, Caers I, et al: Risperidone in the treatment of psychosis of Alzheimer disease: results from a prospective clinical trial. Am J Geriatr Psychiatry 14(3):280–291, 2006 16505133*

Mintzer JE, Tune LE, Breder CD, et al: Aripiprazole for the treatment of psychoses in institutionalized patients with Alzheimer dementia: a multicenter, randomized, double-blind, placebo-controlled assessment of three fixed doses. Am J Geriatr Psychiatry 15(11):918–931, 2007 17974864*

Mohamed S, Rosenheck R, Lyketsos CG, et al: Effect of second-generation antipsychotics on caregiver burden in Alzheimer's disease. J Clin Psychiatry 73(1):121–128, 2012 21939611

Moretti R, Torre P, Antonello RM, et al: Olanzapine as a possible treatment of behavioral symptoms in vascular dementia: risks of cerebrovascular events. A controlled, open-label study. J Neurol 252(10):1186–1193, 2005 15809822*

Mowla A, Pani A: Comparison of topiramate and risperidone for the treatment of behavioral disturbances of patients with Alzheimer disease: a double-blind, randomized clinical trial. J Clin Psychopharmacol 30(1):40–43, 2010 20075646*

Mrak RE, Griffin WS: Dementia with Lewy bodies: Definition, diagnosis, and pathogenic relationship to Alzheimer's disease. Neuropsychiatr Dis Treat 3(5):619–625, 2007 19300591

Mulsant BH, Pollock BG: Psychopharmacology, in The American Psychiatric Publishing Textbook of Geriatric Psychiatry, Fifth Edition. Edited by Steffens DC, Blazer DG, Thakur ME. Arlington, VA, American Psychiatric Publishing, 2015, pp 527–587

Musicco M, Palmer K, Russo A, et al: Association between prescription of conventional or atypical antipsychotic drugs and mortality in older persons with Alzheimer's disease. Dement Geriatr Cogn Disord 31(3):218–224, 2011 21474930*

Ornstein K, Gaugler JE: The problem with "problem behaviors": a systematic review of the association between individual patient behavioral and psychological symptoms and caregiver depression and burden within the dementia patient-caregiver dyad. Int Psychogeriatr 24(10):1536–1552, 2012 22612881

O'Rourke HM, Duggleby W, Fraser KD, Jerke L: Factors that affect quality of life from the perspective of people with dementia: a metasynthesis. J Am Geriatr Soc 63(1):24–38, 2015 25597556

Overall JE, Gorham DR: The Brief Psychiatric Rating Scale (BPRS): recent developments in ascertainment and scaling. Psychopharmacol Bull 24:97–99, 1988

Paleacu D, Barak Y, Mirecky I, Mazeh D: Quetiapine treatment for behavioural and psychological symptoms of dementia in Alzheimer's disease patients: a 6-week, double-blind, placebo-controlled study. Int J Geriatr Psychiatry 23(4):393–400, 2008 17879256*

Pariente A, Fourrier-Reglat A, Ducruet T, et al: Antipsychotic use and myocardial infarction in older patients with treated dementia. Arch Intern Med 172(8):648–653; discussion 654–655, 2012*

Partnership to Improve Dementia Care in Nursing Homes: Antipsychotic drug use in nursing homes trend update. Available at: https://www.nhqualitycampaign.org/files/AP_package_20150421.pdf. Accessed October 2015.

Percudani M, Barbui C, Fortino I, et al: Second-generation antipsychotics and risk of cerebrovascular accidents in the elderly. J Clin Psychopharmacol 25(5):468–470, 2005 16160623*

Pharmacy Quality Alliance (PQA): Technical specifications for PQA approved measures. Springfield, VA, Pharmacy Quality Alliance (PQA), September 2014. 56 p. Available at: http://www.qualitymeasures.ahrq.gov/browse/by-organization-indiv.aspx?orgid=2491&objid=47489. Accessed July 14, 2015.

Pieper MJ, van Dalen-Kok AH, Francke AL, et al: Interventions targeting pain or behaviour in dementia: a systematic review. Ageing Res Rev 12(4):1042–1055, 2013 23727161

Piersanti M, Capannolo M, Turchetti M, et al: Increase in mortality rate in patients with dementia treated with atypical antipsychotics: a cohort study in outpatients in Central Italy. Riv Psichiatr 49(1):34–40, 2014 24572582*

Pijnenburg YA, Sampson EL, Harvey RJ, et al: Vulnerability to neuroleptic side effects in frontotemporal lobar degeneration. Int J Geriatr Psychiatry 18(1):67–72, 2003 12497558

Plassman BL, Langa KM, Fisher GG, et al: Prevalence of dementia in the United States: the aging, demographics, and memory study. Neuroepidemiology 29(1-2):125–132, 2007 17975326

Pollock BG, Mulsant BH, Rosen J, et al: A double-blind comparison of citalopram and risperidone for the treatment of behavioral and psychotic symptoms associated with dementia. Am J Geriatr Psychiatry 15(11):942–952, 2007 17846102*

Pratt NL, Roughead EE, Ramsay E, et al: Risk of hospitalization for stroke associated with antipsychotic use in the elderly: a self-controlled case series. Drugs Aging 27(11):885–893, 2010 20964462*

Pratt N, Roughead EE, Ramsay E, et al: Risk of hospitalization for hip fracture and pneumonia associated with antipsychotic prescribing in the elderly: a self-controlled case-series analysis in an Australian health care claims database. Drug Saf 34(7):567–575, 2011 21663332*

Pressman PS, Miller BL: Diagnosis and management of behavioral variant frontotemporal dementia. Biol Psychiatry 75(7):574–581, 2014 24315411

Prince M, Bryce R, Albanese E, et al: The global prevalence of dementia: a systematic review and metaanalysis. Alzheimers Dement. 9(1):63–75 e62, 2013

Rafaniello C, Lombardo F, Ferrajolo C, et al: Predictors of mortality in atypical antipsychotic-treated community-dwelling elderly patients with behavioural and psychological symptoms of dementia: a prospective population-based cohort study from Italy. Eur J Clin Pharmacol 70(2):187–195, 2014 24145814*

Rainer M, Haushofer M, Pfolz H, et al: Quetiapine versus risperidone in elderly patients with behavioural and psychological symptoms of dementia: efficacy, safety and cognitive function. Eur Psychiatry 22(6):395–403, 2007 17482432*

Richter T, Meyer G, Möhler R, Köpke S: Psychosocial interventions for reducing antipsychotic medication in care home residents. Cochrane Database Syst Rev 12:CD008634, 2012 DOI: 10.1002/14651858.CD008634.pub2 23235663

Rochon PA, Normand SL, Gomes T, et al: Antipsychotic therapy and short-term serious events in older adults with dementia. Arch Intern Med 168(10):1090–1096, 2008 18504337*

Rochon PA, Gruneir A, Gill SS, et al: Older men with dementia are at greater risk than women of serious events after initiating antipsychotic therapy. J Am Geriatr Soc 61(1):55–61, 2013 23301833*

Ropacki SA, Jeste DV: Epidemiology of and risk factors for psychosis of Alzheimer's disease: a review of 55 studies published from 1990 to 2003. Am J Psychiatry 162(11):2022–2030, 2005 16263838

Rosenberg PB, Mielke MM, Han D, et al: The association of psychotropic medication use with the cognitive, functional, and neuropsychiatric trajectory of Alzheimer's disease. Int J Geriatr Psychiatry 27(12):1248–1257, 2012 22374884*

Rosenheck RA, Leslie DL, Sindelar JL, et al; Clinical Antipsychotic Trial of Intervention Effectiveness-Alzheimer's Disease (CATIE-AD) investigators: Cost-benefit analysis of second-generation antipsychotics and placebo in a randomized trial of the treatment of psychosis and aggression in Alzheimer disease. Arch Gen Psychiatry 64(11):1259–1268, 2007 17984395

Rossom RC, Rector TS, Lederle FA, Dysken MW: Are all commonly prescribed antipsychotics associated with greater mortality in elderly male veterans with dementia? J Am Geriatr Soc 58(6):1027–1034, 2010 20487081*

Rountree SD, Chan W, Pavlik VN, et al: Factors that influence survival in a probable Alzheimer disease cohort. Alzheimers Res Ther 4(3):16, 2012 22594761*

Ruths S, Straand J, Nygaard HA, et al: Effect of antipsychotic withdrawal on behavior and sleep/wake activity in nursing home residents with dementia: a randomized, placebo-controlled, double-blinded study. The Bergen District Nursing Home Study. J Am Geriatr Soc 52(10):1737–1743, 2004 15450054*

Ruths S, Straand J, Nygaard HA, Aarsland D: Stopping antipsychotic drug therapy in demented nursing home patients: a randomized, placebo-controlled study—the Bergen District Nursing Home Study (BEDNURS). Int J Geriatr Psychiatry 23(9):889–895, 2008 18306150*

Sacchetti E, Trifirò G, Caputi A, et al: Risk of stroke with typical and atypical anti-psychotics: a retrospective cohort study including unexposed subjects. J Psychopharmacol 22(1):39–46, 2008 18187531*

Sacchetti E, Turrina C, Cesana B, Mazzaglia G: Timing of stroke in elderly people exposed to typical and atypical antipsychotics: a replication cohort study after the paper of Kleijer, et al. J Psychopharmacol 24(7):1131–1132, 2010 19304861*

Savaskan E, Schnitzler C, Schröder C, et al: Treatment of behavioural, cognitive and circadian rest-activity cycle disturbances in Alzheimer's disease: haloperidol vs. quetiapine. Int J Neuropsychopharmacol 9(5):507–516, 2006 16316485*

Savva GM, Zaccai J, Matthews FE, et al; Medical Research Council Cognitive Function and Ageing Study: Prevalence, correlates and course of behavioural and psychological symptoms of dementia in the population. Br J Psychiatry 194(3):212–219, 2009 19252147

Schmedt N, Garbe E: Antipsychotic drug use and the risk of venous thromboembolism in elderly patients with dementia. J Clin Psychopharmacol 33(6):753–758, 2013 24052055*

Schneeweiss S, Setoguchi S, Brookhart A, et al: Risk of death associated with the use of conventional versus atypical antipsychotic drugs among elderly patients. CMAJ 176(5):627–632, 2007 17325327*

Schneider LS, Dagerman KS, Insel P: Risk of death with atypical antipsychotic drug treatment for dementia: meta-analysis of randomized placebo-controlled trials. JAMA 294(15):1934–1943, 2005 16234500

Schneider LS, Tariot PN, Dagerman KS, et al; CATIE-AD Study Group: Effectiveness of atypical antipsychotic drugs in patients with Alzheimer's disease. N Engl J Med 355(15):1525–1538, 2006 17035647*

Selbæk G, Engedal K, Bergh S: The prevalence and course of neuropsychiatric symptoms in nursing home patients with dementia: a systematic review. J Am Med Dir Assoc 14(3):161–169, 2013 23168112

Setoguchi S, Wang PS, Brookhart MA, et al: Potential causes of higher mortality in elderly users of conventional and atypical antipsychotic medications. J Am Geriatr Soc 56(9):1644–1650, 2008 18691283

Shekelle P, Maglione M, Bagley S, et al: Comparative Effectiveness of Off-Label Use of Atypical Antipsychotics. Comparative Effectiveness Review No. 6. (Prepared by the Southern California/RAND Evidence-based Practice Center under Contract No. 290-02-0003.) Rockville, MD, Agency for Healthcare Research and Quality, January 2007. Available at: www.effectivehealthcare.ahrq.gov/reports/final.cfm.

Shiffman RN, Dixon J, Brandt C, et al: The GuideLine Implementability Appraisal (GLIA): development of an instrument to identify obstacles to guideline implementation. BMC Med Inform Decis Mak 5:23, 2005 16048653

Simoni-Wastila L, Ryder PT, Qian J, et al: Association of antipsychotic use with hospital events and mortality among Medicare beneficiaries residing in long-term care facilities. Am J Geriatr Psychiatry 17(5):417–427, 2009 19390299*

Sloane PD, Zimmerman S, Suchindran C, et al: The public health impact of Alzheimer's disease, 2000-2050: potential implication of treatment advances. Annu Rev Public Health 23:213–231, 2002 11910061

Steinberg M, Shao H, Zandi P, et al; Cache County Investigators: Point and 5-year period prevalence of neuropsychiatric symptoms in dementia: the Cache County Study. Int J Geriatr Psychiatry 23(2):170–177, 2008 17607801

Sterke CS, van Beeck EF, van der Velde N, et al: New insights: dose-response relationship between psychotropic drugs and falls: a study in nursing home residents with dementia. J Clin Pharmacol 52(6):947–955, 2012 21628599*

Stinton C, McKeith I, Taylor JP, et al: Pharmacological management of Lewy Body Dementia: A systematic review and meta-analysis. Am J Psychiatry 172(8):731–742, 2015 26085043

Street JS, Clark WS, Gannon KS, et al; The HGEU Study Group: Olanzapine treatment of psychotic and behavioral symptoms in patients with Alzheimer disease in nursing care facilities: a double-blind, randomized, placebo-controlled trial. Arch Gen Psychiatry 57(10):968–976, 2000 11015815*

Streim JE, Porsteinsson AP, Breder CD, et al: A randomized, double-blind, placebo-controlled study of aripiprazole for the treatment of psychosis in nursing home patients with Alzheimer disease. Am J Geriatr Psychiatry 16(7):537–550, 2008 18591574*

Suh GH, Son HG, Ju YS, et al: A randomized, double-blind, crossover comparison of risperidone and haloperidol in Korean dementia patients with behavioral disturbances. Am J Geriatr Psychiatry 12(5):509–516, 2004 15353389*

Suh GH, Greenspan AJ, Choi SK: Comparative efficacy of risperidone versus haloperidol on behavioural and psychological symptoms of dementia. Int J Geriatr Psychiatry 21(7):654–660, 2006 16821257*

Sultana J, Chang CK, Hayes RD, et al: Associations between risk of mortality and atypical antipsychotic use in vascular dementia: a clinical cohort study. Int J Geriatr Psychiatry 29(12):1249–1254, 2014 24633896*

Sultzer DL, Davis SM, Tariot PN, et al; CATIE-AD Study Group: Clinical symptom responses to atypical antipsychotic medications in Alzheimer's disease: phase 1 outcomes from the CATIE-AD effectiveness trial. Am J Psychiatry 165(7):844–854, 2008 18519523*

Tam-Tham H, Cepoiu-Martin M, Ronksley PE, et al: Dementia case management and risk of long-term care placement: a systematic review and meta-analysis. Int J Geriatr Psychiatry 28(9):889–902, 2013 23188735

Tariot PN, Schneider L, Katz IR, et al: Quetiapine treatment of psychosis associated with dementia: a double-blind, randomized, placebo-controlled clinical trial. Am J Geriatr Psychiatry 14(9):767–776, 2006 16905684*

Teranishi M, Kurita M, Nishino S, et al: Efficacy and tolerability of risperidone, yokukansan, and fluvoxamine for the treatment of behavioral and psychological symptoms of dementia: a blinded, randomized trial. J Clin Psychopharmacol 33(5):600–607, 2013 23948783*

Thyrian JR, Eichler T, Hertel J, et al: Burden of behavioral and psychiatric symptoms in people screened positive for dementia in primary care: results of the DelpHi-Study. J Alzheimers Dis 46(2):451–459, 2015 25765916

Trifirò G, Verhamme KM, Ziere G, et al: All-cause mortality associated with atypical and typical antipsychotics in demented outpatients. Pharmacoepidemiol Drug Saf 16(5):538–544, 2007 17036366*

Trifirò G, Gambassi G, Sen EF, et al: Association of community-acquired pneumonia with antipsychotic drug use in elderly patients: a nested case-control study. Ann Intern Med 152(7):418–425, 2010 20368647*

van der Lee J, Bakker TJ, Duivenvoorden HJ, Dröes RM: Multivariate models of subjective caregiver burden in dementia: a systematic review. Ageing Res Rev 15:76–93, 2014 24675045

van Reekum R, Clarke D, Conn D, et al: A randomized, placebo-controlled trial of the discontinuation of long-term antipsychotics in dementia. Int Psychogeriatr 14(2):197–210, 2002 12243210*

Vasilyeva I, Biscontri RG, Enns MW, et al: Movement disorders in elderly users of risperidone and first generation antipsychotic agents: a Canadian population-based study. PLoS ONE 8(5):e64217, 2013 23696870*

Ventura J, Lukoff D, Nuechterlein KH, et al: Training and quality assurance with the Brief Psychiatric Rating Scale. Int J Methods Psychiatr Res 3:221–244, 1993

Verhey FR, Verkaaik M, Lousberg R; Olanzapine-Haloperidol in Dementia Study group: Olanzapine versus haloperidol in the treatment of agitation in elderly patients with dementia: results of a randomized controlled double-blind trial. Dement Geriatr Cogn Disord 21(1):1–8, 2006 16244481*

Vigen CL, Mack WJ, Keefe RS, et al: Cognitive effects of atypical antipsychotic medications in patients with Alzheimer's disease: outcomes from CATIE-AD. Am J Psychiatry 168(8):831–839, 2011 21572163*

Volicer L, Bass EA, Luther SL: Agitation and resistiveness to care are two separate behavioral syndromes of dementia. J Am Med Dir Assoc 8(8):527–532, 2007 17931577

Wallace J, Paauw DS: Appropriate prescribing and important drug interactions in older adults. Med Clin North Am 99(2):295–310, 2015 25700585

Wang PS, Schneeweiss S, Avorn J, et al: Risk of death in elderly users of conventional vs. atypical antipsychotic medications. N Engl J Med 353(22):2335–2341, 2005 16319382*

Wilson RS, Weir DR, Leurgans SE, et al: Sources of variability in estimates of the prevalence of Alzheimer's disease in the United States. Alzheimers Dement 7(1):74–79, 2011 21255745

Woolcott JC, Richardson KJ, Wiens MO, et al: Meta-analysis of the impact of 9 medication classes on falls in elderly persons. Arch Intern Med 169(21):1952–1960, 2009 19933955

Wooten JM: Pharmacotherapy considerations in elderly adults. South Med J 105(8):437–445, 2012 22864103

World Health Organization: Dementia: a public health priority, 2012. Available at: http://www.who.int/mental_health/publications/dementia_report_2012/en/. Accessed May 10, 2015.

Yager J, Kunkle R, Fochtmann LJ, et al: Who's your expert? Use of an expert opinion survey to inform development of American Psychiatric Association practice guidelines. Acad Psychiatry 38(3):376–382, 2014 24493361

Zheng L, Mack WJ, Dagerman KS, et al: Metabolic changes associated with second-generation antipsychotic use in Alzheimer's disease patients: the CATIE-AD study. Am J Psychiatry 166(5):583–590, 2009 19369318

Zhong KX, Tariot PN, Mintzer J, et al: Quetiapine to treat agitation in dementia: a randomized, double-blind, placebo-controlled study. Curr Alzheimer Res 4(1):81–93, 2007 17316169*

# Disclosures

The Guideline Writing Group and Systematic Review Group reported the following disclosures during development and approval of this guideline:

Dr. Reus is employed as a professor of psychiatry at the University of California, San Francisco School of Medicine. He is chairman of the board of the Accreditation Council for Continuing Medical Education (ACCME). He receives travel funds from the ACCME and the American Board of Psychiatry and Neurology (ABPN) for board meetings and test development. He receives research grant support from the National Institute of Mental Health (NIMH) and National Institute on Drug Abuse and honoraria for NIMH grant review service. He reports no conflicts of interest with his work on this guideline.

Dr. Fochtmann is employed as a professor of psychiatry, pharmacological sciences, and biomedical informatics at Stony Brook University. She consults for the American Psychiatric Association on the development of practice guidelines and has received travel funds to attend meetings related to these duties. She has also received travel funds from the American Psychiatric Association to attend the FOCUS self-assessment editorial board meeting. She has received honoraria for serving as a member of NIMH grant review panels, Technical Expert Panels for AHRQ, and Patient-Centered Outcomes Research Institute reviews related to psychiatric topics. She has also received honoraria to present at a meeting of the International Society for ECT and Neurostimulation. She reports no conflicts of interest with her work on this guideline.

Dr. Eyler is employed as a professor of psychiatry and family medicine at the University of Vermont College of Medicine in Burlington, Vermont, and as an attending psychiatrist at the University of Vermont Medical Center and its affiliated hospitals. During the period of preparation of this guideline, honoraria have been received from the University of Vermont College of Medicine, Simmons College, Dartmouth-Hitchcock Medical Center, Dartmouth College, Franklin Pierce University, Greater Manchester [NH] Mental Health Center, and the New Hampshire Department of Corrections. He has provided clinical consultation on gender dysphoria to the department of corrections of the state of New Hampshire, and general psychiatric consultation at The Health Center, a federally qualified health center in Plainfield, Vermont. He is a member of the advisory committee of the Samara Fund, a philanthropic group serving the LGBT communities in Vermont. He has received fees or royalties from Johns Hopkins University Press, Taylor & Francis, and Healthwise, Inc. Travel funds have been provided by the American Psychiatric Association, related to service on the Assembly Executive Committee. He reports no conflicts of interest with his work on this guideline.

Dr. Hilty is employed as a professor of psychiatry at the University of Southern California. He reports no conflicts of interest with his work on this guideline.

Dr. Horvitz-Lennon is employed as a physician scientist at the RAND Corporation and a professor at the Pardee RAND Graduate School. She reports no conflicts of interest with her work on this guideline.

Dr. Jibson is employed as a professor of psychiatry at the University of Michigan. He receives royalties from Up-To-Date for chapters on first- and second-generation antipsychotic medications. He receives grant support and travel funds from the American Board of Psychiatry and Neurology through a Faculty Innovation Fellowship to study the ABPN-mandated Clinical Skills Evaluation in residency programs. He reports no conflicts of interest with his work on this guideline.

Dr. Lopez is employed as a professor of neurology at University of Pittsburgh. He has been principal investigator and co-investigator for research funded by the National Institute on Aging (NIA). He has been the site principal investigator in multicenter trials sponsored by Avid Radiopharmaceuticals, Eli Lilly and Company, Élan, and NIA, and he has received travel funds to attend meetings related to these clinical trials. Dr. Lopez has received consulting fees from H. Lundbeck A/S and Grifols S.A., and he has received travel funds to attend meetings related to this activity. Dr. Lopez has actively participated in the discussions of the creation of all the items of the guideline. However, because his involvement with the industry and government can be perceived as a conflict of interest, he decided to abstain from voting in Statements 7–15 of the guideline.

Dr. Mahoney is employed as a researcher and clinical nurse specialist at The Menninger Clinic in Houston, Texas. She is also an associate professor in the Department of Psychiatry and Behavioral Sciences at Baylor College of Medicine. Dr. Mahoney receives salary support and travel funds from the Arthur Vining Davis Foundations. She reports no conflicts of interest with her work on this guideline.

Dr. Pasic is employed as a professor of psychiatry at the University of Washington. She is a member of the board of the American Association of Emergency Psychiatry. She reports no conflicts of interest with her work on this guideline.

Dr. Tan is employed as an associate professor of geriatric medicine at the David Geffen School of Medicine, University of California, Los Angeles. He receives publication/writing honoraria from WebMD and has received a speaking honorarium from Optimum Health Education. He reports no conflicts of interest with his work on this guideline.

Dr. Wills is employed as an assistant professor of psychiatry at University Hospitals, Case Medical Center. She also has a private practice in forensic psychiatry. She receives no royalties from any entity. She receives travel funds but no honoraria from the American Academy of Psychiatry and the Law. She provides medicolegal consultation and expert testimony to courts. She reports no conflicts of interest with her work on this guideline.

Dr. Rhoads was employed as an assistant professor of psychiatry at the University of Arizona and as a Medical Director for the University of Arizona Medical Center, South Campus, and the Crisis Response Center (CRC) while consulting for the APA on the development of the practice guideline. He subsequently was employed by ConnectionsAZ, continuing as Medical Director of the CRC. He is currently employed as the chief medical officer for Cenpatico Integrated Care, and he is also employed by Correct Care Solutions to perform evaluations in the jail. He reports no conflicts of interest with his work on this guideline.

Dr. Yager is employed as a professor of psychiatry at the University of Colorado. He reports no conflicts of interest with his work on this guideline.

# Individuals and Organizations That Submitted Comments

Vimal M. Aga, M.D.
Rebecca M. Allen, M.D., M.P.H.
James A. Bourgeois, O.D., M.D.
Ryan Carnahan, Pharm.D., BCPP
Lisa K. Catapano-Friedman, M.D.
Huai Y. Cheng, M.D.
Gregory Day, M.D.
D.P. Devanand, M.D.
Brian Draper, M.B.B.S., M.D.
Janel Draxler, R.N., PMHNP
Mary Ann Forciea, M.D.
Norman L. Foster, M.D.
Oliver Freudenreich, M.D.
Wolfang Gaebel, M.D.
Daron Gersch, M.D.
David Goen, R.N., PMHNP
William M. Greenberg, M.D.
Elizabeth Hames, D.O.
Nathan Herrmann, M.D.
Sheila Horras, R.N.
Marilyn Horvath, M.D.
Lee Hyer, Ph.D.
Elie Isenberg-Grzeda, M.D., C.M.
Sefi Knoble, M.D.
Thomas Krajewski, M.D.
John Krystal, M.D.
Amy M. Lewitz, R.N., C.S.
Dinesh Mittal, M.D.
Victor Molinari, Ph.D.

Maureen C. Nash, M.D.
Irene Ortiz, M.D.
David Osser, M.D.
L. Russell Pet, M.D.
Kemuel Philbrick, M.D.
Peter V. Rabins, M.D., M.P.H.
Ryann Rathbone, R.N., PMHNP
Susan Scanland, CRNP, GNP-BC, CDP
Erich Schmidt, Pharm.D., BCPP
Lon S. Schneider, M.D.
Scott Simpson, M.D., M.P.H.
Monica Tegeler, M.D.
Ladislav Volicer, M.D., Ph.D.
Bradley R. Williams, Pharm.D., CGP
Zhan Yang, FNP, PMHNP

APA Council on Geriatric Psychiatry
APA Council on Psychosomatic Medicine
Academy of Psychosomatic Medicine
Alzheimer's Association
American Academy of Family Physicians
American College of Physicians
American Geriatrics Society
American Medical Directors Association—
   The Society for Post-Acute and Long-Term
   Care Medicine
American Psychiatric Nurses Association
American Psychological Association
World Psychiatric Association

# APPENDIX A

# Review of Available Evidence

## Clinical Questions

Evidence review for this guideline was premised on the following clinical questions:

1A. What is the efficacy and comparative effectiveness of second-generation ("atypical") antipsychotics for the treatment of overall behavioral symptoms in patients with Alzheimer's disease and other dementias?
   *Sub-question:* How do second-generation antipsychotic medications compare with other drugs, including first-generation antipsychotics, for the treatment of overall behavioral symptoms?

1B. What are the efficacy and comparative effectiveness of second-generation antipsychotics for the treatment of agitation in patients with Alzheimer's disease and other dementias?
   *Sub-question:* How do second-generation antipsychotic medications compare with other drugs, including first-generation antipsychotics, for the treatment of agitation in patients with Alzheimer's disease and other dementias?

1C. What are the efficacy and comparative effectiveness of second-generation antipsychotics for the treatment of psychosis in patients with Alzheimer's disease and other dementias?
   *Sub-question:* How do second-generation antipsychotic medications compare with other drugs, including first-generation antipsychotics, for the treatment of psychosis in patients with Alzheimer's disease and other dementias?

2. What are the effective dose and time limit for the use of second-generation antipsychotics for the treatment of agitation, psychosis, or overall behavioral symptoms in patients with Alzheimer's disease and other dementias?

3. What subset of patients with Alzheimer's disease and other dementias would potentially benefit from the use of second-generation antipsychotics for the treatment of agitation, psychosis, or overall behavioral symptoms? Do effectiveness and harms differ by race/ethnicity, gender, and age group? by severity of condition and clinical subtype?

4. What are the potential adverse effects and/or complications involved with prescribing of second-generation antipsychotics to patients with Alzheimer's disease and other dementias for the treatment of agitation, psychosis, or overall behavioral symptoms? How do the potential adverse effects and/or complications compare within the class and with other drugs used?

## Review of Supporting Research Evidence

Research evidence related to these clinical questions relies on the 2011 systematic review and meta-analysis conducted by AHRQ on off-label uses of atypical antipsychotic agents (Maglione et al. 2011), which built on a prior AHRQ review (Shekelle et al. 2007). A subsequent systematic review of the literature was conducted by APA staff (see section "Systematic Review Methodology" earlier in this guideline), and ratings of the risk of bias and the quality of the body of research evidence were completed by the Systematic Review Group (see section "Rating the Strength of Supporting Research Evidence" in "Guideline Development Process" earlier in this guideline).

Randomized placebo-controlled trials with sufficient data for standardized mean difference (SMD) calculations of outcome measures were included in the 2011 AHRQ review (Maglione et al. 2011); reported SMD values and summary statistics are from the AHRQ meta-analysis and use Hedges' g to calculate effect size. Jadad scores of evidence quality (Jadad et al. 1996), which range from a low of 0 to a high of 5, were also taken from the AHRQ review when available or determined by the APA Systematic Review Group.

On the basis of the randomized placebo-controlled efficacy trials, the AHRQ report authors concluded that "aripiprazole, olanzapine, and risperidone have efficacy as treatment for behavioral symptoms of dementia" (Maglione et al., 2011, p. ES-5). The same medications were also noted in the AHRQ report to be superior to placebo for the treatment of agitation, with risperidone superior to placebo for the treatment of psychotic symptoms. However, the report authors also found that the "effect sizes were generally considered to be 'small' in magnitude" (Maglione et al. 2011, p. ES-5).

TABLE A–1. Research evidence for efficacy of second-generation antipsychotics (SGAs) from placebo-controlled trials

| Antipsychotic | Symptom domain | Confidence | Effect | SMD (95% CI) |
| --- | --- | --- | --- | --- |
| Aripiprazole | BPSD | Moderate | Small | 0.20 (0.04, 0.35) |
| Aripiprazole | Agitation | Low | Small | — |
| Aripiprazole | Psychosis | Low | Nonsignificant | 0.14 (−0.02, 0.29) |
| Olanzapine | Overall BPSD | Low | Very small | 0.12 (0.00, 0.25) |
| Olanzapine | Agitation | Moderate | Very small | 0.10 (0.07, 0.31) |
| Olanzapine | Psychosis | Insufficient | Nonsignificant | 0.05 (−0.07, 0.17) |
| Quetiapine | Overall BPSD | Low | Nonsignificant | 0.13 (−0.03, 0.28) |
| Quetiapine | Agitation | Insufficient | Nonsignificant | 0.06 (−0.14, 0.25) |
| Quetiapine | Psychosis | Insufficient | Nonsignificant | 0.04 (−0.11, 0.19) |
| Risperidone | Overall BPSD | Moderate | Very small | 0.19 (0.00, 0.38) |
| Risperidone | Agitation | Moderate | Small | 0.22 (0.09, 0.35) |
| Risperidone | Psychosis | Moderate | Small | 0.20 (0.05, 0.36) |
| SGAs overall | Overall BPSD | High | Very small | — |
| SGAs overall | Agitation | Moderate | Small | — |
| SGAs overall | Psychosis | Low | Very small | — |

*Note.* BPSD=behavioral and psychological symptoms of dementia; CI=confidence interval; SMD=standardized mean difference.
*Source.* Adapted from Maglione et al. 2011.

**TABLE A–2.** Research evidence for efficacy from comparator and discontinuation trials

| Comparison | Symptom domain | Confidence | Effect |
| --- | --- | --- | --- |
| SGA vs. haloperidol | Overall BPSD | Low | No difference |
| SGA vs. haloperidol | Agitation | Low | No difference |
| SGA vs. haloperidol | Psychosis | Insufficient | Unable to determine |
| Olanzapine or quetiapine vs. risperidone | Overall BPSD | Low | No difference |
| Olanzapine or quetiapine vs. risperidone | Agitation | Low | No difference |
| Olanzapine or quetiapine vs. risperidone | Psychosis | Insufficient | Unable to determine |
| SGA vs. other comparators | Overall BPSD | Insufficient | Unable to determine |
| SGA vs. other comparators | Agitation | Insufficient | Unable to determine |
| SGA vs. other comparators | Psychosis | Insufficient | Unable to determine |
| Lower doses vs. higher doses | | Insufficient | Unable to determine |
| Continue on antipsychotic vs. change to placebo | | Moderate | Small benefit for continued antipsychotic |

*Note.* BPSD=behavioral and psychological symptoms of dementia; SGA=second-generation antipsychotic.
*Source.* Adapted from Maglione et al. 2011.

In reviewing the adverse effects of antipsychotics in individuals with dementia, the authors of the 2011 AHRQ report (Maglione et al. 2011) compiled evidence from randomized clinical trials in dementia, including the CATIE-AD trial. These studies were primarily placebo-controlled trials; the number of head-to-head trials was relatively small, with few studies on each of the specific comparisons. In general, when compared with placebo, antipsychotics as a class were associated with a greater risk for multiple types of adverse events. In summarizing the strength of evidence for adverse effects of antipsychotics, the authors of the AHRQ report also considered studies of disorders other than dementia in adults of all ages.

Since the 2011 AHRQ report, published data have come from observational studies using large populations of patients from community or health care settings. Data were typically from administrative databases or electronic health records or from follow-up of patients enrolled in clinical services for the treatment of dementia. Other studies used broader populations of individuals 65 years and older in nursing facilities. Although these studies were not restricted to subjects with a diagnosis of dementia, it is likely that a sizeable proportion of individuals with dementia were included in the sample. Many of the studies compared effects of classes of medications (e.g., first-generation vs. second-generation antipsychotic agents, antipsychotic vs. no antipsychotic), but some studies examined effects for specific commonly used antipsychotic agents (e.g., haloperidol, risperidone). Reported outcomes also differed among the studies. Detailed summary statistics were not calculated given these differences in study populations, methodology, and reported outcomes.

# 1A. Efficacy and Comparative Effectiveness of Second-Generation Antipsychotics for Overall BPSD

## Second-Generation Antipsychotic Versus Placebo

### Overview and Quality of Individual Studies

#### Aripiprazole

TABLE A–3. Overview of studies comparing aripiprazole with placebo for treating overall BPSD

| Study type | Study | How subjects were recruited and what intervention(s) were performed[a] | Sample size[b] | How long subjects were followed | Outcome measures and main results | Rating of quality of evidence |
|---|---|---|---|---|---|---|
| 1A | Breder et al. 2004; Mintzer et al. 2007 | Nursing home residents with MMSE scores 6–22 and NPI or NPI-NH score>5 for hallucinations and delusions *Interventions:* placebo and three fixed doses of aripiprazole (2 mg, 5 mg, 10 mg) *Design:* double-blind randomized controlled trial Industry-sponsored multicenter trial conducted in long-term care facilities internationally, including the United States and Canada | 487 subjects enrolled; data for 284 were analyzed | 10 weeks | Aripiprazole vs. placebo: total SMD=0.16 (−0.05, 0.37); psychosis SMD=0.24 (0.03, 0.45); agitation SMD= 0.31 (0.10, 0.52) | 1, 2 |
| 1A | De Deyn et al. 2005 | Non-institutionalized subjects with Alzheimer's disease and psychosis *Interventions:* placebo and aripiprazole at doses ranging from 2 to 15 mg/day (average dose: 10 mg/ day) *Design:* double-blind randomized controlled trial Industry-sponsored multicenter trial conducted in the United States, Canada, Western Europe, and Australia/New Zealand | 208 subjects; 83% completed the trial with no difference in dropouts between placebo and aripiprazole | 10 weeks | Aripiprazole vs. placebo: total SMD=0.06 (−0.21, 0.34); psychosis SMD=0.16 (−0.12, 0.43) | 3 |

| Study type | Study | How subjects were recruited and what intervention(s) were performed[a] | Sample size[b] | How long subjects were followed | Outcome measures and main results | Rating of quality of evidence |
|---|---|---|---|---|---|---|
| 1A | Streim et al. 2008 | Subjects with Alzheimer's disease, residing in nursing homes, with psychosis *Interventions:* placebo, aripiprazole at doses ranging from 0.7 to 15 mg/day (average dose: 8.6 mg/day) *Design:* double-blind randomized controlled trial Industry-sponsored multicenter trial conducted in long-term care facilities in the United States | 256 subjects enrolled; data for 151 were analyzed | 10 weeks, after 1-week washout | Aripiprazole vs. placebo: total SMD=0.36 (0.11, 0.61); psychosis SMD= −0.02 (−0.27, 0.23); agitation SMD= 0.30 (0.05, 0.55) | 2 |

*Note.* 1=randomized controlled trial; 2=systematic review/meta-analysis; 3=observational; A=from AHRQ review. AHRQ=Agency for Healthcare Research and Quality; BPSD=behavioral and psychological symptoms of dementia; MMSE=Mini-Mental State Examination; NPI=Neuropsychiatric Inventory; NPI-NH=Neuropsychiatric Inventory—Nursing Home; SMD = standardized mean difference.
[a]Includes additional notes that may impact quality rating.
[b]Where applicable. Note overall *N* as well as group *n* for control and intervention.

### Quality of the Body of Research Evidence for Aripiprazole Versus Placebo for Overall BPSD

*Risk of bias:* **Low**—Studies are all RCTs and are primarily of moderate quality based on their described randomization and blinding procedures and their descriptions of study dropouts.

*Consistency:* **Consistent**—Effect sizes are overlapping and have the same magnitude and direction of effect.

*Directness:* **Direct**—Studies measure overall BPSD, which is directly related to the PICOTS questions.

*Precision:* **Imprecise**—Confidence intervals are relatively narrow, but the range of confidence intervals includes negative values in two of the three studies.

*Applicability:* The included studies all involve individuals with dementia, with two of the studies involving nursing home or hospital patients and one study involving non-institutionalized patients. The studies include subjects from around the world, including the United States, Canada, Western Europe, and Australia/New Zealand. The doses of aripiprazole that were used in the studies are consistent with usual practice.

*Dose-response relationship:* **Absent**—A single study examined the effect of different doses of aripiprazole relative to placebo. Although examination of confidence intervals suggests a tendency for a dose response, these dose-response relationships did not show statistical differences across each pair of doses.

*Magnitude of effect:* **Weak**—The effect size is relatively small.

*Confounding factors:* **Absent**—No known confounding factors are present that would be likely to reduce the effect of the intervention.

*Publication bias:* **Not suspected**—There is no specific evidence to suggest selection bias.

*Overall strength of evidence:* **Moderate**—The three available studies of aripiprazole vs. placebo are randomized trials of low to moderate quality and have good sample sizes. However, there is some variability in the confidence intervals and no clear dose-response relationships.

## Olanzapine

**TABLE A–4.** **Overview of studies comparing olanzapine with placebo for treating overall BPSD**

| Study type | Study | How subjects were recruited and what intervention(s) were performed[a] | Sample size[b] | How long subjects were followed | Outcome measures and main results | Rating of quality of evidence |
|---|---|---|---|---|---|---|
| 1A | Deberdt et al. 2005 | Subjects with Alzheimer's dementia, vascular dementia, or mixed dementia, in outpatient or residential settings, with NPI or NPI-NH score>5 on hallucination and delusion items<br>*Interventions:* placebo vs. flexibly dosed olanzapine (2.5–10 mg/day; mean dose: 5.2 mg/day) or risperidone (0.5–2 mg/day; mean dose: 1.0 mg/day)<br>*Design:* double-blind randomized trial<br>Industry-sponsored multicenter trial in the United States | 494 subjects, with 94 receiving placebo, 204 receiving olanzapine, and 196 receiving risperidone | 10 weeks | Olanzapine vs. placebo: total SMD=−0.02 (−0.27, 0.23); psychosis SMD=−0.12(−0.36,0.13); agitation SMD=0.09 (−0.16, 0.34) | 2 |
| 1A | De Deyn et al. 2004 | Subjects with Alzheimer's disease (MMSE scores 5–26), in long-term care settings, with hallucinations or delusions<br>*Interventions:* placebo or fixed doses of olanzapine (1, 2.5, 5, or 7.5 mg/day)<br>*Design:* double-blind randomized trial in Europe, Israel, Lebanon, Australia/New Zealand, and South Africa<br>Industry-sponsored multicenter trial | 652 subjects; 65%–75% of subjects in each study arm completed the trial | 10 weeks | Olanzapine vs. placebo: total SMD=0.14 (−0.05, 0.34); psychosis SMD = 0.17 (−0.02, 0.37); agitation SMD=0.14 (−0.05, 0.33) | 2 |

**Overview of studies comparing olanzapine with placebo for treating overall BPSD** *(continued)*

| Study type | Study | How subjects were recruited and what intervention(s) were performed[a] | Sample size[b] | How long subjects were followed | Outcome measures and main results | Rating of quality of evidence |
|---|---|---|---|---|---|---|
| 1A | Schneider et al. 2006; Sultzer et al. 2008 | Subjects with Alzheimer's disease or probable Alzheimer's disease (MMSE scores 5–26), ambulatory and residing at home or in assisted living, with moderate or greater levels of psychosis, aggression, or agitation *Interventions:* placebo vs. masked, flexibly dosed olanzapine (mean dose: 5.5 mg/day), quetiapine (mean dose: 56.5 mg/day), or risperidone (mean dose: 1.0 mg/day) Stable doses of cholinesterase inhibitor were permitted. *Design:* multicenter, federally funded CATIE-AD trial—Phase 1 | 421 subjects randomly assigned to treatment group, with 142 receiving placebo, 100 receiving olanzapine, 94 receiving quetiapine, and 85 receiving risperidone | Median duration on Phase 1 treatment was 7.1 weeks; clinical outcomes assessed for those continuing to receive antipsychotic at 12 weeks | Olanzapine vs. placebo: total SMD=0.15 (−0.11, 0.40); psychosis SMD=0.07 (−0.19, 0.33); agitation SMD=0.28 (0.02, 0.53) | 1 |
| 1A | Street et al. 2000 | Subjects with possible or probable Alzheimer's disease, residing in a nursing facility, with NPI-NH score >2 *Interventions:* placebo vs. fixed doses of olanzapine (5, 10, or 15 mg/day) *Design:* double-blind randomized controlled trial Industry-sponsored multicenter trial in the United States | 206 subjects; 66%–80% of subjects in each study arm completed the trial | 6 weeks | Olanzapine vs. placebo: total SMD=0.30 (−0.03, 0.63); psychosis SMD= 0.17 (−0.17, 0.50); agitation SMD=0.39 (0.05, 0.72) | 5 |

*Note.* 1=randomized controlled trial; 2=systematic review/meta-analysis; 3=observational; A=from AHRQ review.
AHRQ=Agency for Healthcare Research and Quality; BPSD=behavioral and psychological symptoms of dementia; CATIE-AD=Clinical Antipsychotic Trials of Intervention Effectiveness for Alzheimer's Disease; MMSE=Mini-Mental State Examination; NPI = Neuropsychiatric Inventory; NPI-NH=Neuropsychiatric Inventory—Nursing Home; SMD=standardized mean difference.
[a]Includes additional notes that may impact quality rating.
[b]Where applicable. Note overall *N* as well as group *n* for control and intervention.

*Quality of the Body of Research Evidence for Olanzapine Versus Placebo for Overall BPSD*

*Risk of bias:* **Low**—Studies are all RCTs and vary in quality from low to high quality based on their described randomization and blinding procedures and their descriptions of study dropouts.

*Consistency:* **Consistent**—Effect sizes are overlapping and have the same magnitude. Three of the four studies show the same direction of effect, with the fourth study showing no effect.

*Directness:* **Direct**—Studies measure overall BPSD, which is directly related to the PICOTS questions.

*Precision:* **Imprecise**—Confidence intervals are relatively narrow, but the range of confidence intervals includes negative values in all four studies.

*Applicability:* The included studies all involve individuals with dementia, with three of the studies involving nursing home or hospital patients and two of the studies involving non-institutionalized patients. The studies include subjects from around the world, including the United States, Western Europe, and Australia/New Zealand. The doses of olanzapine that were used in the studies are consistent with usual practice.

*Dose-response relationship:* **Absent**—Two studies examined different doses of olanzapine and showed opposite effects. One showed improved response at higher doses, whereas the other study showed improved response at lower doses.

*Magnitude of effect:* **Weak**—The effect size is quite small and barely statistically significant.

*Confounding factors:* **Absent**—No known confounding factors are present that would be likely to reduce the effect of the intervention.

*Publication bias:* **Not suspected**—There is no specific evidence to suggest selection bias.

*Overall strength of evidence:* **Low**—The available studies of olanzapine versus placebo are randomized trials and have good sample sizes, but the trials are of varying quality and the imprecise nature of the results and the clear lack of a dose-response effect reduce confidence in the findings.

# Quetiapine

**TABLE A–5.** Overview of studies comparing quetiapine with placebo for treating overall BPSD

| Study type | Study | How subjects were recruited and what intervention(s) were performed[a] | Sample size[b] | How long subjects were followed | Outcome measures and main results | Rating of quality of evidence |
|---|---|---|---|---|---|---|
| 1A | Schneider et al. 2006; Sultzer et al. 2008 | Subjects with Alzheimer's disease or probable Alzheimer's disease (MMSE scores 5–26), ambulatory and residing at home or in assisted living, with moderate or greater levels of psychosis, aggression, or agitation<br>*Interventions:* placebo vs. masked, flexibly dosed olanzapine (mean dose: 5.5 mg/day), quetiapine (mean dose: 56.5 mg/day), or risperidone (mean dose: 1.0 mg/day)<br>Stable doses of cholinesterase inhibitor were permitted.<br>*Design:* multicenter, federally funded CATIE-AD trial—Phase 1 | 421 subjects randomly assigned to treatment group, with 142 receiving placebo, 100 receiving olanzapine, 94 receiving quetiapine, and 85 receiving risperidone | Median duration on Phase 1 treatment was 7.1 weeks; clinical outcomes assessed for those who continued to take antipsychotic at 12 weeks | Quetiapine vs. placebo: total SMD= 0.15 (−0.11, 0.42); psychosis SMD= 0.16 (−0.10, 0.42); agitation SMD= 0.10 (−0.17, 0.37) | 1 |
| 1A | Tariot et al. 2006 | Subjects with Alzheimer's disease meeting criteria for DSM-IV (MMSE score>4), residing in a nursing facility, with psychosis and BPRS score>23<br>*Interventions:* placebo vs. flexibly dosed haloperidol (0.5–12 mg/day; median of the mean daily dose: 1.9 mg) or quetiapine (25–600 mg/day; median of the mean daily dose: 96.9 mg)<br>*Design:* double-blind randomized controlled trial<br>Industry-sponsored multicenter trial in the United States | 284 subjects; data for 180 were analyzed | 10 weeks | Quetiapine vs. placebo: total SMD= 0.22 (−0.07, 0.28); psychosis SMD= 0.00 (−0.29, 0.30); agitation SMD= 0.24 (−0.05, 0.54) | 4 |

**Overview of studies comparing quetiapine with placebo for treating overall BPSD** *(continued)*

| Study type | Study | How subjects were recruited and what intervention(s) were performed[a] | Sample size[b] | How long subjects were followed | Outcome measures and main results | Rating of quality of evidence |
|---|---|---|---|---|---|---|
| 1A | Zhong et al. 2007 | Subjects with possible Alzheimer's disease or vascular dementia, in long-term care facilities, with agitation and PANSS-EC score>13 *Interventions:* placebo vs. quetiapine 100 mg vs. quetiapine 200 mg (dose adjusted according to fixed titration) *Design:* double-blind randomized trial Industry-sponsored multicenter trial in the United States | 333 subjects | 10 weeks | Quetiapine vs. placebo: total SMD= 0.04 (−0.21, 0.28); psychosis SMD= −0.03 (−0.27, 0.21); agitation SMD= −0.03 (−0.27, 0.21) | 2 |

*Note.* 1=randomized controlled trial; 2=systematic review/meta-analysis; 3=observational; A=from AHRQ review. AHRQ=Agency for Healthcare Research and Quality; BPRS=Brief Psychiatric Rating Scale; BPSD=behavioral and psychological symptoms of dementia; CATIE-AD=Clinical Antipsychotic Trials of Intervention Effectiveness for Alzheimer's Disease; MMSE=Mini-Mental State Examination; PANSS-EC=Positive and Negative Symptom Scale—Excitement Component; SMD=standardized mean difference.
[a]Includes additional notes that may impact quality rating.
[b]Where applicable. Note overall $N$ as well as group $n$ for control and intervention.

### Quality of the Body of Research Evidence for Quetiapine Versus Placebo for Overall BPSD

*Risk of bias:* **Low**—Studies are all RCTs and vary in quality from low to high quality based on their described randomization and blinding procedures and their descriptions of study dropouts.

*Consistency:* **Consistent**—Effect sizes in the meta-analysis are overlapping and have the same size. The three studies in the meta-analysis show the same direction of effect, but in none of the studies is the effect statistically significant. In addition, the overall effect in the meta-analysis is not statistically significant. The fourth study shows an improvement in the Clinical Global Impressions (CGI), which is consistent with a beneficial overall effect.

*Directness:* **Direct**—Studies measure overall BPSD, which is directly related to the PICOTS questions.

*Precision:* **Imprecise**—Confidence intervals are relatively narrow, but the range of confidence intervals includes negative values in all the studies included in the meta-analysis.

*Applicability:* The included studies all involve individuals with dementia, with two of the studies involving nursing home or hospital patients and one study involving non-institutionalized patients. An additional study did not specify the setting where the subjects were recruited. The studies include subjects from the United States. The doses of quetiapine that were used in the studies are consistent with usual practice.

*Dose-response relationship:* **Absent**—One study examined differing doses of quetiapine and showed no effect at either dose.

*Magnitude of effect:* **Weak effect**—The effect size is quite small and not statistically significant.

*Confounding factors:* **Absent**—No known confounding factors are present that would be likely to reduce the effect of the intervention.

*Publication bias:* **Not suspected**—There is no specific evidence to suggest selection bias.

*Overall strength of evidence:* **Low**—The available studies of quetiapine versus placebo are randomized trials of varying quality. Three of the five studies have good sample sizes, and the confidence intervals are relatively narrow. However, the lack of precision and the absence of a dose-response effect suggest less confidence in the findings.

## Risperidone

**TABLE A–6.** **Overview of studies comparing risperidone with placebo for treating overall BPSD**

| Study type | Study | How subjects were recruited and what intervention(s) were performed[a] | Sample size[b] | How long subjects were followed | Outcome measures and main results | Rating of quality of evidence |
|---|---|---|---|---|---|---|
| 1A | Brodaty et al. 2003, 2005 | Subjects with DSM-IV diagnosis of dementia of the Alzheimer's type, vascular dementia, or mixed dementia, residing in nursing homes, with MMSE score <24 and significant aggressive behavior<br>*Interventions:* placebo vs. risperidone (flexibly dosed up to 2 mg/day; mean dose: 0.95 mg/day).<br>*Design:* double-blind randomized trial<br>Industry-sponsored multicenter trial in Australia/New Zealand | 345 subjects | 12 weeks | Risperidone vs. placebo: total SMD= 0.46 (0.23, 0.69); psychosis SMD= 0.36 (0.13, 0.59); agitation SMD= 0.37 (0.14, 0.59) | 3 |
| 1A | Deberdt et al. 2005 | Subjects with Alzheimer's dementia, vascular dementia, or mixed dementia, in outpatient or residential settings, with NPI or NPI-NH score >5 on hallucination and delusion items<br>*Interventions:* placebo vs. flexibly dosed olanzapine (2.5–10 mg/day; mean dose: 5.2 mg/day) or risperidone (0.5–2 mg/day; mean dose: 1.0 mg/day)<br>*Design:* double-blind randomized trial<br>Industry-sponsored multicenter trial in the United States | 494 subjects, with 94 receiving placebo, 204 receiving olanzapine, and 196 receiving risperidone | 10 weeks | Risperidone vs. placebo: total SMD= −0.13 (−0.38, 0.12); psychosis SMD= −0.03 (−0.34, 0.16); agitation SMD= 0.14 (−0.11, 0.39) | 2 |

| Study type | Study | How subjects were recruited and what intervention(s) were performed[a] | Sample size[b] | How long subjects were followed | Outcome measures and main results | Rating of quality of evidence |
|---|---|---|---|---|---|---|
| 1A | De Deyn et al. 1999 | Hospitalized or institutionalized subjects with MMSE score<24 and BEHAVE-AD score>7 *Interventions:* placebo vs. flexibly dosed haloperidol (0.5–4 mg/day; mean dose: 1.2 mg/day) or risperidone (0.5–4 mg/day; mean dose: 1.1 mg/day) *Design:* randomized trial Industry-sponsored multicenter trial in the United Kingdom and Europe | 344 subjects; 68 of 115 subjects treated with risperidone, 81 of 115 subjects treated with haloperidol, and 74 of 114 subjects receiving placebo completed the trial | 12 weeks | Risperidone vs. placebo: total SMD= 0.12 (−0.14, 0.38); agitation SMD= 0.31 (0.05, 0.57) | 4 |
| 1A | Katz et al. 1999 | Subjects with DSM-IV diagnosis of Alzheimer's disease, vascular dementia, or mixed dementia, residing in a nursing home or chronic care facility, with MMSE score <24 and significant psychotic and behavioral symptoms (BEHAVE-AD score>7) *Interventions:* placebo vs. fixed doses of risperidone (0.5 mg/day, 1 mg/day, or 2 mg/day) *Design:* double-blind randomized controlled trial Industry-sponsored multicenter trial conducted in the United States | 625 subjects; 70% of whom completed the study | 12 weeks | Risperidone vs. placebo: total SMD= 0.32 (0.11, 0.53); psychosis SMD= 0.20 (−0.01, 0.41); agitation SMD= 0.38 (0.17, 0.60) | 4 |
| 1A | Mintzer et al. 2006 | Subjects with symptoms meeting criteria for Alzheimer's dementia (MMSE scores 5–23), residing in nursing homes or long-term care facilities, who were mobile and had psychosis *Interventions:* placebo vs. flexibly dosed risperidone (0.5–1.5 mg/day; mean dose: 1.03 mg/day) *Design:* randomized controlled trial Industry-sponsored multicenter trial conducted in the United States | 473 subjects randomly assigned to treatment group, with 238 receiving placebo and 235 receiving risperidone; 354 of the subjects completed the study | 8 weeks, after 1–16 days of placebo run-in/ washout | Risperidone vs. placebo: total SMD= −0.01 (−0.21, 0.18); psychosis SMD= 0.17 (−0.02, 0.36); agitation SMD= 0.04 (−0.16, 0.23) | 3 |

**Overview of studies comparing risperidone with placebo for treating overall BPSD** *(continued)*

| Study type | Study | How subjects were recruited and what intervention(s) were performed[a] | Sample size[b] | How long subjects were followed | Outcome measures and main results | Rating of quality of evidence |
|---|---|---|---|---|---|---|
| 1A | Schneider et al. 2006; Sultzer et al. 2008 | Subjects with Alzheimer's disease or probable Alzheimer's disease (MMSE scores 5–26), ambulatory and residing at home or in assisted living, with moderate or greater levels of psychosis, aggression, or agitation<br>*Interventions:* placebo vs. masked, flexibly dosed olanzapine (mean dose: 5.5 mg/day), quetiapine (mean dose: 56.5 mg/day), or risperidone (mean dose: 1.0 mg/day)<br>Stable doses of cholinesterase inhibitor were permitted.<br>*Design:* multicenter, federally funded CATIE-AD trial—Phase 1 | 421 subjects randomly assigned to treatment group, with 142 receiving placebo, 100 receiving olanzapine, 94 receiving quetiapine, and 85 receiving risperidone | Median duration on Phase 1 treatment was 7.1 weeks; clinical outcomes assessed for those continuing to receive antipsychotic at 12 weeks | Risperidone vs. placebo: total SMD= 0.40 (0.13, 0.68); psychosis SMD= 0.38 (0.11, 0.66); agitation SMD= 0.10 (−0.17, 0.37) | 1 |

*Note.* 1=randomized controlled trial; 2=systematic review/meta-analysis; 3=observational; A=from AHRQ review. AHRQ=Agency for Healthcare Research and Quality; BEHAVE-AD=Behavioral Pathology in Alzheimer's Disease; BPSD=behavioral and psychological symptoms of dementia; CATIE-AD=Clinical Antipsychotic Trials of Intervention Effectiveness for Alzheimer's Disease; MMSE=Mini-Mental State Examination; NPI=Neuropsychiatric Inventory; NPI-NH=Neuropsychiatric Inventory—Nursing Home; SMD=standardized mean difference.
[a]Includes additional notes that may impact quality rating.
[b]Where applicable. Note overall $N$ as well as group $n$ for control and intervention.

### Quality of the Body of Research Evidence for Risperidone Versus Placebo for Overall BPSD

*Risk of bias:* **Low**—Studies are all RCTs and vary in quality from low to high quality based on their described randomization and blinding procedures and their descriptions of study dropouts.

*Consistency:* **Inconsistent**—Effect sizes are generally overlapping but vary in direction, with four studies showing an effect in the direction of risperidone benefit, one study showing no effect, and one study showing an effect in the direction of benefit for placebo. Three of the four studies showing a benefit of risperidone were statistically significant, but the other three studies did not show statistically significant benefit.

*Directness:* **Direct**—Studies measure overall BPSD, which is directly related to the PICOTS questions.

*Precision:* **Imprecise**—Confidence intervals are relatively narrow, but the range of confidence intervals includes negative values in three of the six studies.

*Applicability:* The included studies all involve individuals with dementia, with four of the studies involving nursing home or hospital patients and two of the studies involving non-institutionalized patients. The studies include subjects from around the world, including the United States, United Kingdom, Western Europe, and Australia/New Zealand. The doses of risperidone that were used in the studies are consistent with usual practice.

Quetiapine Versus Haloperidol

**TABLE A–8.** **Overview of studies comparing quetiapine with haloperidol for treating overall BPSD**

| Study type | Study | How subjects were recruited and what intervention(s) were performed[a] | Sample size[b] | How long subjects were followed | Outcome measures and main results | Rating of quality of evidence |
|---|---|---|---|---|---|---|
| 1A | Savaskan et al. 2006 | Inpatients with ICD-10 Alzheimer's disease and associated behavioral symptoms<br>*Interventions:* haloperidol (0.5–4 mg/day; mean dose: 1.9 mg/day) vs. quetiapine (25–200 mg/day; mean dose: 125 mg/day); fixed titration schedule with weekly dose increments to final dose<br>*Design:* randomized controlled open-label trial<br>Trial conducted in Switzerland; two of the three investigators were noted to be supported by an industry-sponsored grant. | 30 subjects enrolled; 4 dropped out, and 4 had missing data; data for 22 were analyzed | 5 weeks, after run-in period of up to 7 days | Quetiapine vs. haloperidol: total SMD=0.99 (0.10, 1.88); agitation SMD=0.06 (−0.78, 0.89) | 2 |
| 1A | Tariot et al. 2006 | Subjects with DSM-IV Alzheimer's disease (MMSE score>4), residing in nursing facilities, with psychosis and BPRS score>23<br>*Interventions:* placebo vs. flexibly dosed haloperidol (0.5–12 mg/day; mean dose: 1.9 mg/day) or quetiapine (25–600 mg/day; mean dose: 96.9 mg/day)<br>*Design:* double-blind randomized controlled trial<br>Industry-sponsored multicenter trial in the United States | 284 subjects; data for 180 were analyzed | 10 weeks | Quetiapine vs. haloperidol: total SMD=0.16 (−0.16, 0.47); agitation SMD=0.04 (−0.26, 0.34) | 4 |

*Note.* 1=randomized controlled trial; 2=systematic review/meta-analysis; 3=observational; A=from AHRQ review.
AHRQ=Agency for Healthcare Research and Quality; BPSD=behavioral and psychological symptoms of dementia; MMSE=Mini-Mental State Exam; SMD=standardized mean difference.
[a]Includes additional notes that may impact quality rating.
[b]Where applicable. Note overall $N$ as well as group $n$ for control and intervention.

**TABLE A–9.** Overview of studies comparing risperidone with haloperidol for treating overall BPSD

| Study type | Study | How subjects were recruited and what intervention(s) were performed[a] | Sample size[b] | How long subjects were followed | Outcome measures and main results | Rating of quality of evidence |
|---|---|---|---|---|---|---|
| 1 | Chan et al. 2001 | Inpatients or outpatients with DSM-IV diagnosis of dementia of Alzheimer's type or vascular dementia associated with behavioral symptoms. *Interventions:* flexibly dosed haloperidol (0.5–2 mg/day; mean dose: 0.90 mg/day) vs. risperidone (0.5–2 mg/day; mean dose: 0.85 mg/day). *Design:* double-blind randomized controlled trial. Industry-sponsored multicenter trial conducted in Hong Kong | 58 subjects | 3 months | Haloperidol vs. risperidone: change in BEHAVE-AD dementia (aggressiveness): SMD = 0.057 (−0.472, 0.585); change in BEHAVE-AD dementia (psychosis): SMD = −0.383 (−0.917, 0.15) Scores on the CMAI and BEHAVE-AD were significantly improved by both haloperidol and risperidone, with no significant differences between the two treatments. Patients treated with haloperidol, but not those treated with risperidone, showed an increase in EPS on the SAS. | 3 |
| 1A | De Deyn et al. 1999 | Hospitalized or institutionalized subjects with MMSE score <24 and BEHAVE-AD score >7. *Interventions:* placebo vs. flexibly dosed haloperidol (0.5–4 mg/day; mean dose: 1.2 mg/day) or risperidone (0.5–4 mg/day; mean dose: 1.1 mg/day). *Design:* randomized trial. Industry-sponsored multicenter trial in the United Kingdom and Europe | 344 subjects; 68 of the 115 subjects treated with risperidone, 81 of the 115 subjects treated with haloperidol, and 74 of the 114 subjects receiving placebo completed the trial | 12 weeks | Risperidone vs. haloperidol: total SMD = −0.19 (−0.45, 0.07); agitation SMD = −0.07 (−0.19, −0.33) | 4 |

**Overview of studies comparing risperidone with haloperidol for treating overall BPSD** *(continued)*

| Study type | Study | How subjects were recruited and what intervention(s) were performed[a] | Sample size[b] | How long subjects were followed | Outcome measures and main results | Rating of quality of evidence |
|---|---|---|---|---|---|---|
| 1 | Suh et al. 2004, 2006 | Subjects in a nursing facility with a diagnosis of Alzheimer's disease, vascular dementia, or mixed dementia associated with behavioral disturbance FAST>3, BEHAVE-AD score>7, and CMAI score>2 on at least two items<br><br>*Interventions:* flexibly dosed risperidone (0.5–1.5 mg/day; mean dose: 0.80 mg/day) vs. haloperidol (0.5–1.5 mg/day; mean dose: 0.83 mg/day)<br><br>*Design:* randomized double-blind crossover trial<br>Industry-sponsored trial at a single center in Korea | 120 | 18 weeks | Compared with treatment with haloperidol, risperidone treatment was associated with greater clinical improvement on total and subscale scores of the Korean version of BEHAVE-AD, total and subscale scores of the Korean version of CMAI, and the CGI-C as well as a lower frequency of EPS. | 4 |

*Note.* 1=randomized controlled trial; 2=systematic review/meta-analysis; 3=observational; A=from AHRQ review. AHRQ=Agency for Healthcare Research and Quality; BEHAVE-AD=Behavioral Pathology in Alzheimer's Disease; BPSD=behavioral and psychological symptoms of dementia; CGI-C=Clinical Global Impression of Change; CMAI= Cohen-Mansfield Agitation Inventory; EPS=extrapyramidal side effects; FAST=Functional Assessment Staging; MMSE=Mini-Mental State Exam; SAS=Simpson-Angus Scale; SMD=standardized mean difference.
[a]Includes additional notes that may impact quality rating.
[b]Where applicable. Note overall $N$ as well as group $n$ for control and intervention.

## Quality of the Body of Research Evidence for Second-Generation Antipsychotics Versus Haloperidol for Overall BPSD

*Risk of bias:* **Low**—Studies are all RCTs and vary in quality from low to high quality based on their described randomization and blinding procedures and their descriptions of study dropouts.

*Consistency:* **Inconsistent**—Effect sizes are inconsistent for trials of the same medication as well as across the body of comparisons. Several of the studies have an extremely wide confidence interval.

*Directness:* **Direct**—Studies measure overall BPSD, which is directly related to the PICOTS questions.

*Precision:* **Imprecise**—Confidence intervals are variable in width, and several confidence intervals are extremely wide.

*Applicability:* The included studies all involve individuals with dementia, with seven of the studies including nursing home or hospital patients and two studies including non-institutionalized patients. The studies include subjects from around the world, including the United States, Western Europe, Korea, and Hong Kong. The doses of haloperidol and SGA that were used in the studies are consistent with usual practice.

*Dose-response relationship:* **Not applicable for this comparison.**

*Magnitude of effect:* **Not applicable.**

*Confounding factors:* **Absent**—No known confounding factors are present that would be likely to reduce the effect of the intervention.

*Publication bias:* **Not suspected**—There is no specific evidence to suggest selection bias.

*Overall strength of evidence:* **Low**—The available studies of SGA medications as compared with haloperidol include six randomized parallel arm trials and one randomized crossover trial, but the trials are of varying quality and some have small sample sizes. For the five trials that were included in the AHRQ meta-analysis, the effect size is small and does not show evidence of a difference between haloperidol and SGAs overall. For individual agents, there are no more than two studies for each drug, and several of the studies have extremely wide confidence intervals.

## Overview and Quality of Individual Studies

TABLE A–10. **Overview of studies comparing olanzapine or quetiapine with risperidone for treating overall BPSD**

| Study type | Study | How subjects were recruited and what intervention(s) were performed[a] | Sample size[b] | How long subjects were followed | Outcome measures and main results | Rating of quality of evidence |
|---|---|---|---|---|---|---|
| 1A | Deberdt et al. 2005 | Subjects with Alzheimer's dementia, vascular dementia, or mixed dementia, in outpatient or residential settings, with NPI or NPI-NH score>5 on hallucination and delusion items *Interventions:* placebo vs. flexibly dosed olanzapine (2.5–10 mg/day; mean dose: 5.2 mg/day) or risperidone (0.5–2 mg/day; mean dose: 1.0 mg/day) *Design:* double-blind randomized trial Industry-sponsored multicenter trial in the United States | 494 subjects, with 94 receiving placebo, 204 receiving olanzapine, and 196 receiving risperidone | 10 weeks | Olanzapine vs. risperidone: total SMD=0.10 (−0.10, 0.30); psychosis SMD=−0.03 (−0.23, 0.17); agitation SMD= −0.04 (−0.24, 0.16) | 2 |
| 1 | Fontaine et al. 2003 | Subjects with DSM-IV diagnosis of dementia in long-term care facilities in the United States *Interventions:* olanzapine (2.5–10 mg/day; mean dose: 6.65 mg/day) vs. risperidone (0.5–2 mg/day; mean dose: 1.47 mg/day) *Design:* double-blind parallel study | 39 subjects, with 20 receiving olanzapine and 19 receiving risperidone | 2 weeks | Both risperidone and olanzapine were associated with significant decreases in CGI-C and NPI scores ($P<0.0001$) and an improved score on a quality-of-life measure (Quality of Life in Late Stage Dementia) ($P<0.03$), however, the drugs did not differ in the magnitude of their effects on these measures. The most common adverse events were drowsiness and falls. At baseline, 42% (16/38) of subjects had extrapyramidal symptoms, and there was no significant change in SAS scores with treatment. | 3 |

| Study type | Study | How subjects were recruited and what intervention(s) were performed[a] | Sample size[b] | How long subjects were followed | Outcome measures and main results | Rating of quality of evidence |
|---|---|---|---|---|---|---|
| 1 | Gareri et al. 2004 | Subjects with a DSM-IV diagnosis of Alzheimer's disease, vascular dementia, or mixed dementia associated with behavioral symptoms<br>*Interventions:* promazine 50 mg/day vs. risperidone 1 mg/day vs. olanzapine 5 mg/day; doses could be doubled at 4 weeks if no clinical response<br>*Design:* double-blind randomized trial conducted in Western Europe; setting of care not specified | 60 enrolled (20 per group); 1 withdrawal in risperidone group | 8 weeks, after 10-day washout | Global improvement was noted in 80% of patients treated with risperidone and olanzapine and in 65% of patients treated with promazine. | 3 |
| 1A | Schneider et al. 2006; Sultzer et al. 2008 | Subjects with Alzheimer's disease or probable Alzheimer's disease (MMSE scores 5–26), ambulatory and residing at home or in assisted living, with moderate or greater levels of psychosis, aggression, or agitation Stable doses of cholinesterase inhibitor were permitted.<br>*Interventions:* placebo vs. masked, flexibly dosed olanzapine (mean dose: 5.5 mg/day), quetiapine (mean dose: 56.5 mg/day), or risperidone (mean dose: 1.0 mg/day)<br>*Design:* multicenter, federally funded CATIE-AD trial—Phase 1 | 421 subjects randomly assigned to treatment group, with 142 receiving placebo, 100 receiving olanzapine, 94 receiving quetiapine, and 85 receiving risperidone | Median duration on Phase 1 treatment was 7.1 weeks; clinical outcomes assessed for those continuing to receive antipsychotic at 12 weeks | Olanzapine vs. risperidone: total SMD= −0.27 (−0.56, 0.02); psychosis SMD= −0.27 (−0.56, 0.02); agitation SMD=−0.17 (−0.12, 0.16)<br>Quetiapine vs. risperidone: total SMD= −0.24 (−0.53, 0.06); psychosis SMD= −0.24 (−0.54, 0.05); agitation SMD=0.10 (−0.20, 0.39) | 1 |

| Study type | Study | How subjects were recruited and what intervention(s) were performed[a] | Sample size[b] | How long subjects were followed | Outcome measures and main results | Rating of quality of evidence |
|---|---|---|---|---|---|---|
| 1A | Rainer et al. 2007 | Outpatients with mild to moderate dementia of the Alzheimer's, vascular, mixed, or frontotemporal lobe type according to DSM-IV and ICD-10 who had behavioral disturbance and NPI sub-item scores relating to psychosis or agitation/aggression *Interventions:* flexibly dosed quetiapine (50–400 mg/day; mean dose: 77 mg/day) vs. risperidone (0.5–4 mg/day; mean dose: 0.9 mg/day) *Design:* single-blind, parallel-group randomized trial Investigator-sponsored multicenter trial in Western Europe | 72 enrolled, with 65 subjects in ITT population (34 patients receiving quetiapine and 31 patients receiving risperidone) | 8 weeks | Quetiapine vs. risperidone: total SMD= −0.06 (−0.55, 0.43); agitation SMD=−0.17 (−0.66, 0.32) | 3 |

*Note.* 1=randomized controlled trial; 2=systematic review/meta-analysis; 3=observational; A=from AHRQ review. AHRQ=Agency for Healthcare Research and Quality; BPSD=behavioral and psychological symptoms of dementia; CATIE-AD=Clinical Antipsychotic Trials of Intervention Effectiveness for Alzheimer's Disease; CGI-C=Clinical Global Impression of Change; ITT=intention to treat; MMSE=Mini-Mental State Exam; NPI=Neuropsychiatric Inventory; NPI-NH=Neuropsychiatric Inventory—Nursing Home; SAS=Simpson-Angus Scale; SMD=standardized mean difference.
[a]Includes additional notes that may impact quality rating.
[b]Where applicable. Note overall $N$ as well as group $n$ for control and intervention.

## Quality of the Body of Research Evidence for Olanzapine or Quetiapine Versus Risperidone for Overall BPSD

*Risk of bias:* **Low**—Studies are all RCTs but vary in quality from low to moderate based on their described randomization and blinding procedures and their descriptions of study dropouts.

*Consistency:* **Inconsistent**—Effect sizes are overlapping, and the direction of the effect was variable. However, none of the studies, including those that were not part of the AHRQ meta-analysis, show prominent differences between risperidone and either olanzapine or quetiapine.

*Directness:* **Direct**—Studies measure overall BPSD, which is directly related to the PICOTS questions.

*Precision:* **Imprecise**—Confidence intervals are relatively wide, and the range of confidence intervals includes negative values in all four studies.

*Applicability:* The included studies all involve individuals with dementia, including patients in institutional and outpatient settings. The studies include subjects from around the world, including the

United States and Western Europe. The doses of medication that were used in the studies are consistent with usual practice.

*Dose-response relationship:* **Not applicable to this comparison.**

*Magnitude of effect:* **Not applicable.**

*Confounding factors:* **Absent**—No known confounding factors are present that would be likely to reduce the effect of the intervention.

*Publication bias:* **Not suspected**—There is no specific evidence to suggest selection bias.

*Overall strength of evidence:* **Low**—The available studies of risperidone as compared with olanzapine or quetiapine are randomized trials of low to moderate quality. The studies vary in their sample sizes. In addition, several of the confidence intervals are wide. For the four trials that were included in the AHRQ meta-analysis, no overall effect size was calculated, but there does not appear to be evidence of a difference between olanzapine or quetiapine and risperidone for overall BPSD.

## Second-Generation Antipsychotic Versus Other Comparators

### Overview and Quality of Individual Studies

**TABLE A–11. Overview of studies comparing second-generation antipsychotics with other medications for treating overall BPSD**

| Study type | Study | How subjects were recruited and what intervention(s) were performed[a] | Sample size[b] | How long subjects were followed | Outcome measures and main results | Rating of quality of evidence |
|---|---|---|---|---|---|---|
| 1 | Ballard et al. 2005 | Subjects with a diagnosis of Alzheimer's disease, residing in nursing care facilities in England, with clinically significant agitation *Interventions:* placebo vs. rivastigmine (3–6 mg BID by week 12 and >8 mg daily by week 26) vs. quetiapine (25–50 mg BID by week 12 and 50 mg BID by week 26) *Design:* double-blind randomized controlled trial Funded by general donations to the principal investigator's research program and profits from prior industry-sponsored trials | 93 subjects; 80 started treatment (25 receiving rivastigmine, 26 receiving quetiapine, and 29 receiving placebo), and 71 tolerated the maximum protocol dose (22 rivastigmine, 23 quetiapine, 26 placebo); 56 had a baseline score of >10 on the SIB, and 46 of these subjects were included in the analysis at 6-week follow up (14 receiving rivastigmine, 14 receiving quetiapine, and 18 receiving placebo). | 26 weeks total; primary outcome was agitation at 6 weeks | Rivastigmine vs. quetiapine: change in CMAI dementia (agitation) SMD=−0.051 (−0.601, 0.499) When treated with either rivastigmine or quetiapine as compared with placebo, subjects failed to show an improvement in agitation. Relative to placebo, quetiapine, but not rivastigmine, was associated with greater cognitive decline as measured by the SIB score. | 4 |

| Study type | Study | How subjects were recruited and what intervention(s) were performed[a] | Sample size[b] | How long subjects were followed | Outcome measures and main results | Rating of quality of evidence |
|---|---|---|---|---|---|---|
| 1 | Barak et al. 2011 | Inpatients with Alzheimer's dementia who had been admitted for behavioral symptoms, including psychosis and agitation<br>*Interventions:* risperidone 1 mg/day vs. escitalopram 10 mg/day<br>*Design:* double-blind randomized trial<br>Trial conducted in Israel | 40 subjects | 6 weeks | Degree of improvement as measured by the NPI was comparable in those treated with risperidone as compared with those treated with escitalopram. Premature discontinuation occurred in 45% of risperidone-treated subjects and 25% of escitalopram-treated subjects, primarily because of adverse events. Serious adverse effects, including severe extrapyramidal side effects and acute illness requiring hospitalization, occurred in 6 risperidone-treated patients. | 5 |

| Study type | Study | How subjects were recruited and what intervention(s) were performed[a] | Sample size[b] | How long subjects were followed | Outcome measures and main results | Rating of quality of evidence |
|---|---|---|---|---|---|---|
| 1 | Culo et al. 2010 | Subjects with dementia with Lewy body (DLB) or Alzheimer's disease (AD) who were hospitalized for behavioral disturbance<br>*Interventions:* risperidone (started at 0.5 mg/day for 3 days, then increased to two capsules/day for 2 weeks, with two additional dosage increases up to four capsules/day allowed) vs. citalopram (started at 10 mg/day for 3 days, then increased to two capsules/day for 2 weeks, with two additional dosage increases up to four capsules/day allowed)<br>*Design:* double-blind randomized controlled trial<br>Trial conducted at Western Psychiatric Institute and Clinic in Pittsburgh, PA | 31 patients with DLB and 66 patients with AD; of the 408 patients who were prescreened, 111 signed consent and were screened, and 103 were randomly assigned to treatment group | Up to 12 weeks | Efficacy of citalopram or risperidone was comparable for subjects overall, but AD patients showed improved scores on the NPI and CGI-C, whereas DLB patients showed a worsening on both measures. Discontinuation rates were similar for DLB patients who were treated with citalopram (71%) or risperidone (65%). However, premature discontinuation rates were higher in participants with DLB (68%) than in those with AD (50%), and treated DLB subjects who had been randomly assiged to receive risperidone had more side effects. | 4 |

| Study type | Study | How subjects were recruited and what intervention(s) were performed[a] | Sample size[b] | How long subjects were followed | Outcome measures and main results | Rating of quality of evidence |
|---|---|---|---|---|---|---|
| 1 | De Deyn et al. 2012 | Subjects age 65 years or older with Alzheimer's disease, residing in nursing homes or equivalent institutions, with symptoms of psychosis and/or agitation *Interventions:* XR vs. IR quetiapine; doses were 50 mg/day XR and 25 mg/day IR. Treatment was escalated to 100 mg/day by day 4 (for both XR and IR). At day 8, a period of flexible dosing (50–300 mg/day) began when dose adjustment was made at the investigator's discretion *Design:* double-blind, double-dummy, parallel-group randomized controlled trial Trial conducted at 14 sites in Australia, Belgium, Canada, Norway, and South Africa | Of the 109 patients screened, 100 were randomly assigned to receive quetiapine XR ($n=68$) or quetiapine IR ($n=32$); 90 patients completed the study (1 patient receiving quetiapine XR withdrew because of an adverse event). | 6 weeks; enrollment and screening were conducted between May 2002 and February 2003 | Relative to baseline, both the IR and the XR formulations of quetiapine were associated with improvements in NPI frequency x severity total score and the NPI disruption score, as well as improvements in the CMAI score. Global ratings using the CGI–Severity of Illness and CGI–Improvement scores also showed benefit from both formulations. | 3 |

TABLE A–11. **Overview of studies comparing second-generation antipsychotics with other medications for treating overall BPSD** *(continued)*

| Study type | Study | How subjects were recruited and what intervention(s) were performed[a] | Sample size[b] | How long subjects were followed | Outcome measures and main results | Rating of quality of evidence |
|---|---|---|---|---|---|---|
| 1 | Freund-Levi et al. 2014a, 2014b | Subjects with a diagnosis of dementia and associated neuropsychiatric symptoms who were being treated on an inpatient or outpatient basis at a university hospital in Sweden *Interventions:* galantamine (target dose: 24 mg) vs. risperidone (target dose: 1.5 mg) *Design:* open-label randomized trial Trial conducted at a single center in Sweden | 100 subjects (50 in each group); 91 completed the study | 12 weeks | Treatments with galantamine and with risperidone were associated with decreases in agitation. However, improvement was more pronounced with risperidone than with galantamine (mean difference in total CMAI score: 3.7 points at 3 weeks [$P=0.03$] and 4.3 points at 12 weeks [$P=0.01$]). NPI domains of irritation and agitation also showed greater benefit with risperidone ($F_{(1,97)}=5.2$, $P=0.02$). However, galantamine treatment was associated with an improvement in MMSE scores, with an increase of 2.8 points compared with baseline (95% CI: 1.96, 3.52). No severe treatment-related side effects were reported with either treatment. | 0 |

| Study type | Study | How subjects were recruited and what intervention(s) were performed[a] | Sample size[b] | How long subjects were followed | Outcome measures and main results | Rating of quality of evidence |
|---|---|---|---|---|---|---|
| 1A | Holmes et al. 2007 | Subjects with severe probable Alzheimer's disease, residing in nursing home setting, with MMSE score<6 and CMAI score>3 for at least 6 weeks<br>*Interventions:* fixed titration with rivastigmine 3–6 mg/day vs. risperidone 0.5 mg/day<br>Exclusion criteria included prior exposure to cholinesterase inhibitor or antipsychotic (>20 mg thioridazine equivalents per day).<br>*Design:* double-blind randomized controlled trial<br>Trial conducted in the United Kingdom | 27 subjects | 6 weeks | Rivastigmine vs. risperidone: change in CMAI (agitation) SMD= 1.31 (0.47–2.15) | 3 |
| 1 | Mowla and Pani 2010 | Subjects with mild to moderate DSM-IV Alzheimer's disease and behavioral disturbance<br>*Interventions:* flexibly dosed topiramate (average dose: 44 mg/day) or risperidone (average dose: 1.9 mg/day)<br>*Design:* randomized controlled trial<br>Multisite trial; Bushehr University of Medical Sciences, Iran | 48 subjects, with 25 receiving topiramate and 23 receiving risperidone; 41 total subjects completed the trial | 8 weeks | Topiramate vs. risperidone: change in NPI (total) SMD=0.23 (−0.38, 0.85); change in CMAI (agitation) SMD=0.06 (−0.56, 0.67)<br>Both topiramate and risperidone were associated with significant improvements in all outcome measures. | 5 |

**TABLE A-11. Overview of studies comparing second-generation antipsychotics with other medications for treating overall BPSD** *(continued)*

| Study type | Study | How subjects were recruited and what intervention(s) were performed[a] | Sample size[b] | How long subjects were followed | Outcome measures and main results | Rating of quality of evidence |
|---|---|---|---|---|---|---|
| 1 | Pollock et al. 2007 | Subjects with dementia admitted to hospital for moderate to severe agitation or psychosis but no significant depressive symptoms or recent depressive episodes and no unstable physical illness *Interventions:* flexibly dosed citalopram (average dose: 29.4 mg/day) or risperidone (average dose: 1.25 mg/day) Subjects could continue taking cholinesterase inhibitors or memantine if they had been taking them for at least 12 weeks at a stable dose; lorazepam at up to 2 mg/day was also permitted for extreme agitation or aggression. *Design:* Double-blind randomized trial Trial conducted in Canada; funding by U.S. Public Health Service and Sandra A. Rotman Program in Neuropsychiatry, Toronto, Ontario, Canada | 408 subjects were screened; 103 were randomly assigned (citalopram, $n=53$; risperidone, $n=50$); 45 completed treatment (citalopram, $n=25$; risperidone, $n=20$) | 12-week trial conducted between February 2000 to June 2005 | No significant differences were seen between citalopram and risperidone in outcomes or time to dropout. On the NRS, there were significant decreases in psychosis scores for both medications (32.3% and 35.2% decreases for citalopram and risperidone, respectively). The decrease in agitation scores was significant for citalopram (12.5%) but not for risperidone (8.2%). | 5 |

| Study type | Study | How subjects were recruited and what intervention(s) were performed[a] | Sample size[b] | How long subjects were followed | Outcome measures and main results | Rating of quality of evidence |
|---|---|---|---|---|---|---|
| 1 | Teranishi et al. 2013 | Subjects with DSM-IV Alzheimer's dementia admitted to hospital for unmanageable behavioral symptoms <br> *Interventions:* flexibly dosed risperidone (average dose: 1.1 mg/day), yokukansan (average dose: 7 mg/day), or fluvoxamine (average dose: 83 mg/day) <br> Subjects could continue taking donepezil and could receive anticholinergic medications for EPS and zopiclone or brotizolam for insomnia. <br> *Design:* rater-blinded randomized trial <br> Trial conducted at a psychiatric hospital in Japan | 90 subjects screened; 82 enrolled and data for 76 analyzed (risperidone, $n=25$; yokukansan, $n=26$; fluvoxamine, $n=25$) | 8 weeks, preceded by 1-week washout, with data collected between January 2009 and August 2010 | All three drugs significantly reduced NPI-NH total scores from 26.20 (SD, 15.77) to 17.72 (SD, 11.49), with no significant differences among groups. Single-item scores were significantly reduced for delusions, agitation, disinhibition, aberrant motor behavior, and nighttime behavior disturbances, again with no significant group differences. MMSE scores and FIM scores showed no significant change during the study. Constipation was the most common adverse event in all groups, with a significant increase in frequency with risperidone. EPS and muscle rigidity were also significantly increased in frequency with risperidone (19.2% of that treatment group). | 2 |

*Note.* 1=randomized controlled trial; 2=systematic review/meta-analysis; 3=observational; A=from AHRQ review.
AHRQ=Agency for Healthcare Research and Quality; BPSD=behavioral and psychological symptoms of dementia; CATIE-AD=Clinical Antipsychotic Trials of Intervention Effectiveness for Alzheimer's Disease; CGI=Clinical Global Impression; CGI-C=Clinical Global Impression of Change; CI=confidence interval; CMAI=Cohen-Mansfield Agitation Inventory; EPS=extrapyramidal side effects; FIM=Functional Independence Measure; IR=immediate release; MMSE=Mini-Mental State Exam; NPI=Neuropsychiatric Inventory; NPI-NH=Neuropsychiatric Inventory—Nursing Home; NRS=Neurobehavioral Rating Scale; SIB=Severe Impairment Battery; SAS = Simpson-Angus Scale; SD=standard deviation; SMD=standardized mean difference; XR=extended release.
[a]Includes additional notes that may impact quality rating.
[b]Where applicable. Note overall $N$ as well as group $n$ for control and intervention.

## Quality of the Body of Research Evidence for Second-Generation Antipsychotics Versus Other Medications for Overall BPSD

*Risk of bias:* **Moderate**—Studies are all RCTs, but not all are double-blind. The studies also vary in quality from low to high quality based on their described randomization and blinding procedures and their descriptions of study dropouts.

*Consistency:* **Consistent**—Virtually all of the studies show no differences between the two treatment groups.

*Directness:* **Direct**—Studies measure overall BPSD, which is directly related to the PICOTS questions.

*Precision:* **Not applicable**—Confidence intervals are not available for the majority of the studies.

*Applicability:* The included studies all involve individuals with dementia and include subjects in institutional and non-institutional settings. The studies include subjects from around the world, including the United States, Canada, Western Europe, Australia/New Zealand, Iran, and Japan. The doses of medication that were used in the studies are consistent with usual practice.

*Dose-response relationship:* **Not applicable for this comparison.**

*Magnitude of effect:* **Not applicable**—Confidence intervals are not available for the majority of the studies.

*Confounding factors:* **Absent**—No known confounding factors are present that would be likely to reduce the effect of the intervention.

*Publication bias:* **Not suspected**—There is no specific evidence to suggest selection bias.

*Overall strength of evidence:* **Insufficient**—The available studies of SGAs compared with other interventions are highly variable in their quality and sample sizes. Although the majority of the studies use risperidone as an antipsychotic medication, the comparators include an anticonvulsant, cholinesterase inhibitors, and antidepressants, making it difficult to arrive at any overall conclusions from these head-to-head comparisons.

# Discontinuation Studies

## Overview and Quality of Individual Studies

**TABLE A–12. Overview of studies looking at effects of discontinuing antipsychotics compared with placebo**

| Study type | Study | How subjects were recruited and what intervention(s) were performed[a] | Sample size[b] | How long subjects were followed | Outcome measures and main results | Rating of quality of evidence |
|---|---|---|---|---|---|---|
| 1 | Ballard et al. 2004 | Nursing home residents with probable or possible Alzheimer's disease (by NINCDS/ADRDA criteria) who had no severe behavioral disturbances and had been taking neuroleptics for longer than 3 months *Interventions:* prescriptions written, in a twice-daily regimen, allocating the closest dose to participant's preexisting prescription from the doses encapsulated (risperidone 0.5 mg, chlorpromazine 12.5 mg, thioridazine 12.5 mg, trifluoperazine 0.5 mg, haloperidol 0.25 mg) After randomization, study medication replaced existing medication on the day of commencement. *Design:* double-blind, placebo-controlled randomized discontinuation study Multicenter trial in the United Kingdom | 100 subjects enrolled, with 82 completing 1-month assessment (36 receiving placebo, 46 receiving active treatment) | 3 months | Subjects with higher baseline NPI scores ($>14$) were significantly more likely to develop marked behavioral problems when antipsychotic medication was discontinued ($\chi^2=6.8$, $P=0.009$). Similar proportions of antipsychotic- and placebo-treated subjects withdrew from the study prematurely, overall and because of worsening behavioral symptoms. | 3 |

| Study type | Study | How subjects were recruited and what intervention(s) were performed[a] | Sample size[b] | How long subjects were followed | Outcome measures and main results | Rating of quality of evidence |
|---|---|---|---|---|---|---|
| 1 | Ballard et al. 2008, 2009 | Subjects with dementia, residing in nursing facilities, who had been receiving antipsychotic medication for at least 3 months for behavioral or psychiatric disturbance<br>*Interventions:* continuation of antipsychotic (thioridazine, chlorpromazine, haloperidol, trifluoperazine, or risperidone) or change to receiving placebo<br>*Design:* Blinded, placebo-controlled, parallel-group randomized discontinuation trial Multicenter trial (Dementia Antipsychotic Withdrawal Trial) in the United Kingdom | 165 subjects randomly assigned to treatment group (83 to antipsychotic treatment group; 82 to placebo group); 128 initiated intervention (64 in each condition); 13 were lost to follow-up in each study arm. 51 subjects per condition completed the study. | 12 months | Continuation treatment and placebo groups had no significant difference in the estimated mean change between baseline and 6 months in SIB scores (estimated mean difference in deterioration favoring placebo: −0.4 [95% CI: −6.4, 5.5]) or NPI scores (estimated mean difference in deterioration favoring continued treatment: −2.4 [95% CI: −8.2, 3.5]). There continued to be no difference between continuation treatment and placebo groups at 12 months, although some evidence suggested that subjects with initial NPI scores ≥15 showed reduced neuropsychiatric symptoms with continuing treatment. Subjects who continued to receive antipsychotic treatment had a lower cumulative probability of survival at 12 months, with 70% (95% CI: 58%, 80%) survival in the continued treatment group versus 77% (95% CI: 64%, 85%) in the placebo group for subjects receiving at least one dose of drug or placebo. Differences between groups were more pronounced at longer periods of follow-up (24-month survival: 46% vs. 71%; 36-month survival: 30% vs. 59%) with an HR of 0.58 (95% CI: 0.35, 0.95). | 5 |

| Study type | Study | How subjects were recruited and what intervention(s) were performed[a] | Sample size[b] | How long subjects were followed | Outcome measures and main results | Rating of quality of evidence |
|---|---|---|---|---|---|---|
| 1 | Devanand et al. 2011 | Outpatients with Alzheimer's disease with psychosis or agitation who had responded to 20 weeks of open-label haloperidol (0.5–5 mg/day) as defined by a minimum of a 50% reduction in three target symptoms, and improvement in CGI-C score for psychosis/agitation *Interventions:* randomization to placebo vs. continuation of haloperidol *Design:* double-blind randomized trial in the United States | 44 patients at trial entry; of the 22 responders to haloperidol, 21 entered the randomized portion of the trial, and 20 had at least one follow-up visit. | 6 months | Open-label haloperidol was associated with a significant decrease in symptoms but a significant increase in EPS. 4 of 10 patients who continued to take haloperidol relapsed as compared with 8 of 10 patients receiving placebo, but this difference was not statistically significant. (Relapse criteria required 50% worsening in target symptoms and CGI-C scores.) Time to relapse was shorter for placebo than for haloperidol ($P=0.04$). | 3 |

| Study type | Study | How subjects were recruited and what intervention(s) were performed[a] | Sample size[b] | How long subjects were followed | Outcome measures and main results | Rating of quality of evidence |
|---|---|---|---|---|---|---|
| 1 | Devanand et al. 2012 | Patients with Alzheimer's disease and psychosis or agitation-aggression, 50–95 years of age, who were recruited from memory clinics (including Alzheimer's research centers), geriatric psychiatry clinics, and clinics at Veterans Affairs medical centers; through physician referrals and advertising; or from assisted-living facilities (outpatient or residents) or nursing homes *Interventions:* 16-week open-label risperidone phase, then randomization to one of three regimens: continued risperidone therapy for 32 weeks (group 1), risperidone therapy for 16 weeks followed by placebo for 16 weeks (group 2), or placebo for 32 weeks (group 3) *Design:* double-blind randomized controlled trial | 180 patients received open-label risperidone (mean dose, 0.97 mg/day). Criteria for response to treatment were met in 112 patients; 110 of these subjects underwent randomization. | 32 weeks in randomized phase (after the 16-week open-label phase) | Outcome measures: time to relapse of psychosis or agitation, adverse events, mortality. 16-week relapse rate was higher in patients receiving placebo than in those treated with risperidone (60% [24 of 40 patients in group 3] vs. 33% [23 of 70 in groups 1 and 2]; $P=0.004$; HR with placebo=1.94; 95% CI: 1.09, 3.45; $P=0.02$). 32-week relapse rate was higher in group 2 than in group 1 (48% [13 of 27 patients in group 2] vs. 15% [2 of 13 in group 1]; $P=0.02$; HR=4.88; 95% CI: 1.08, 21.98; $P=0.02$). | 5 |
| 1 | Ruths et al. 2004, 2008 | Subjects with dementia, residing in nursing homes, who were taking haloperidol, risperidone, or olanzapine for nonpsychotic symptoms for at least 3 months *Interventions:* continuation of treatment with antipsychotic medication or change to placebo *Design:* double-blind, placebo-controlled randomized trial Multicenter trial in Norway | 55 subjects; 27 of the subjects had antipsychotic medication discontinued, and 28 had antipsychotic medication continued. | 4 weeks | In subjects who had antipsychotic discontinued, the proportion of individuals who continued not to take an antipsychotic medication was 85%, 46%, and 33% at 1, 2, and 5 months after drug discontinuation. In a subset of 30 patients, antipsychotic discontinuation was associated with reduced sleep efficiency and greater activity levels as measured by actigraphy. | 4 |

**Overview of studies looking at effects of discontinuing antipsychotics compared with placebo** *(continued)*

| Study type | Study | How subjects were recruited and what intervention(s) were performed[a] | Sample size[b] | How long subjects were followed | Outcome measures and main results | Rating of quality of evidence |
|---|---|---|---|---|---|---|
| 1 | van Reekum et al. 2002 | Subjects with dementia, residing in nursing facilities, who had been receiving antipsychotic medication (risperidone, olanzapine, haloperidol, thioridazine, or loxapine) for more than 6 months, and had behavioral symptoms that were currently stable<br>*Interventions:* continue treatment or change to placebo<br>*Design:* randomized trial of antipsychotic discontinuation<br>Multicenter trial in Canada; not industry sponsored | 34 subjects; 10 of the 16 subjects receiving placebo and 6 of the 16 subjects receiving active treatment withdrew from the trial before completion. | 6 months | About one-quarter of subjects in each group showed a worsening of behavioral symptoms. More subjects in the placebo group withdrew from the study for worsening behavior, but this difference was not statistically significant. Data suggested that subjects taking a higher baseline dose of antipsychotic were more likely to have a worsening of behavior upon discontinuation of antipsychotic medication. | 3 |

*Note.* 1=randomized controlled trial; 2=systematic review/meta-analysis; 3=observational; A=from AHRQ review. AHRQ=Agency for Healthcare Research and Quality; ADRDA=Alzheimer's Disease and Related Disorders Association; CGI-C=Clinical Global Impression of Change; CI=confidence interval; EPS=extrapyramidal side effects; HR=Kaplan-Meier hazard ratio; NINCDS=National Institute of Neurological and Communicative Diseases; NPI=Neuropsychiatric Inventory; NPI-Q=NPI-Questionnaire; SIB=Severe Impairment Battery.
[a]Includes additional notes that may impact quality rating.
[b]Where applicable. Note overall *N* as well as group *n* for control and intervention.

## Quality of the Body of Research Evidence From Discontinuation Studies in Terms of Overall BPSD

*Risk of bias:* **Low**—All studies use an open-label phase of treatment for stabilization on antipsychotic followed by randomization for the discontinuation portion of the trial. The studies vary in quality from moderate to high quality based on their described randomization and blinding procedures and their descriptions of study dropouts.

*Consistency:* **Consistent**—Although the studies with small samples did not always reach statistical significance, the discontinuation studies consistently showed greater proportions of individuals in the placebo group who withdrew because of worsening of symptoms. Studies that examined the effect of baseline behavioral symptoms showed a greater risk of worsening when subjects who had greater symptoms at baseline had their antipsychotic treatment discontinued.

*Directness:* **Indirect**—Studies measure overall BPSD following discontinuation, which is related to the PICOTS questions.

*Precision:* **Imprecise**—Although confidence intervals are not available for these measures, the lack of statistical significance for these measures in several of the studies indicates uncertainty about the conclusions.

*Applicability:* The included studies all involve individuals with dementia, including nursing home, hospital, and non-institutionalized patients. The studies include subjects from around the world, including the United States, Canada, United Kingdom, and Western Europe. The doses of medication that were used in the studies are consistent with usual practice.

*Dose-response relationship:* **Not applicable.**

*Magnitude of effect:* **Weak**—Effect is measured in terms of worsening symptoms in the placebo group as compared with the group who continued to receive an antipsychotic.

*Confounding factors:* **Absent**—No known confounding factors are present that would be likely to reduce the effect of the intervention.

*Publication bias:* **Not suspected**—There is no specific evidence to suggest selection bias.

*Overall strength of evidence:* **Moderate**—The trials are of good quality overall and consistent in the direction of effects seen, but the variations in the statistical significance of results reduce the level of confidence in the finding.

# 1B. Efficacy and Comparative Effectiveness of Second-Generation Antipsychotics for Treatment of Agitation

## Second-Generation Antipsychotic Versus Placebo

### Overview and Quality of Individual Studies

Aripiprazole

TABLE A–13. **Overview of studies comparing aripiprazole with placebo for treating agitation**

| Study type | Study | How subjects were recruited and what intervention(s) were performed[a] | Sample size[b] | How long subjects were followed | Outcome measures and main results | Rating of quality of evidence |
|---|---|---|---|---|---|---|
| 1A | Breder et al. 2004; Mintzer et al. 2007 | Nursing home residents with MMSE scores 6–22 and NPI or NPI-NH score >5 for hallucinations and delusions *Interventions:* placebo and three fixed doses of aripiprazole (2 mg, 5 mg, 10 mg) *Design:* double-blind randomized controlled trial Industry-sponsored multicenter trial conducted in long-term care facilities internationally, including the United States and Canada | 487 subjects enrolled; data for 284 analyzed | 10 weeks | Aripiprazole vs. placebo: total SMD = 0.16 (−0.05, 0.37); psychosis SMD=0.24 (0.03, 0.45); agitation SMD=0.31 (0.10, 0.52) | 1, 2 |

| Study type | Study | How subjects were recruited and what intervention(s) were performed[a] | Sample size[b] | How long subjects were followed | Outcome measures and main results | Rating of quality of evidence |
|---|---|---|---|---|---|---|
| 1A | Streim et al. 2008 | Nursing home residents with Alzheimer's disease with psychosis<br>*Interventions:* placebo, aripiprazole at 0.7–15 mg/day (average dose: 8.6 mg/day)<br>*Design:* double-blind randomized controlled trial<br>Industry-sponsored multicenter trial conducted in long-term care facilities in the United States | 256 subjects enrolled; data for 151 analyzed | 10 weeks, after 1-week washout | Aripiprazole vs. placebo: total SMD=0.36 (0.11, 0.61); psychosis SMD=−0.02 (−0.27, 0.23); agitation SMD=0.30 (0.05, 0.55) | 2 |

*Note.* 1=randomized controlled trial; 2=systematic review/meta-analysis; 3=observational; A=from AHRQ review.
AHRQ=Agency for Healthcare Research and Quality; MMSE=-Mini Mental State Exam; NPI=Neuropsychiatric Inventory; NPI-NH = Neuropsychiatric Inventory—Nursing Home; SMD=standardized mean difference.
[a]Includes additional notes that may impact quality rating.
[b]Where applicable. Note overall *N* as well as group *n* for control and intervention.

### *Quality of the Body of Research Evidence for Aripiprazole Versus Placebo in Agitation*

*Risk of bias:* **Moderate**—Studies are both RCTs but are of low quality based on their described randomization and blinding procedures and their descriptions of study dropouts.

*Consistency:* **Consistent**—Effect sizes are overlapping, relatively narrow, and in the same direction.

*Directness:* **Direct**—Studies measure agitation, which is directly related to the PICOTS questions.

*Precision:* **Precise**—Confidence intervals are relatively narrow, and the range of confidence intervals does not include negative values.

*Applicability:* The included studies all involve individuals with dementia, with two of the studies including nursing home or hospital patients and one study including non-institutionalized patients. The studies include subjects from the United States and Canada. The doses of aripiprazole that were used in the studies are consistent with usual practice.

*Dose-response relationship:* **Absent**—In the one study that assessed this for agitation, the 5-mg and 10-mg doses of aripiprazole were more effective than the 2-mg dose, although the difference was not statistically significant.

*Magnitude of effect:* **Weak effect**—The effect size is relatively small.

*Confounding factors:* **Absent**—No known confounding factors are present that would be likely to reduce the effect of the intervention.

*Publication bias:* **Not suspected**—There is no specific evidence to suggest selection bias.

*Overall strength of evidence:* **Low**—Only two studies of aripiprazole versus placebo are available that assessed agitation. These have good sample sizes and are randomized trials but are of low to moderate quality.

# Olanzapine

**TABLE A–14. Overview of studies comparing olanzapine with placebo for treating agitation**

| Study type | Study | How subjects were recruited and what intervention(s) were performed[a] | Sample size[b] | How long subjects were followed | Outcome measures and main results | Rating of quality of evidence |
|---|---|---|---|---|---|---|
| 1A | Deberdt et al. 2005 | Subjects with Alzheimer's dementia, vascular dementia, or mixed dementia, in outpatient or residential settings, with NPI or NPI-NH score>5 on hallucination and delusion items<br>*Interventions:* placebo vs. flexibly dosed olanzapine (2.5–10 mg/day; mean dose: 5.2 mg/day) or risperidone (0.5–2 mg/day; mean dose: 1.0 mg/day)<br>*Design:* double-blind randomized trial<br>Industry-sponsored multicenter trial in the United States | 494 subjects, with 94 receiving placebo, 204 receiving olanzapine, and 196 receiving risperidone | 10 weeks | Olanzapine vs. placebo: total SMD=−0.02 (−0.27, 0.23); psychosis SMD=−0.12 (−0.36, 0.13); agitation SMD=0.09 (−0.16, 0.34) | 2 |
| 1A | De Deyn et al. 2004 | Subjects with Alzheimer's disease (MMSE scores 5–26), in long-term care settings, with hallucinations or delusions<br>*Interventions:* placebo or fixed-dose olanzapine (1, 2.5, 5, or 7.5 mg/day)<br>*Design:* double-blind randomized trial<br>Industry-sponsored multicenter trial in Europe, Israel, Lebanon, Australia/New Zealand, and South Africa | 652 subjects; 65%–75% of the subjects in each study arm completed the trial | 10 weeks | Olanzapine vs. placebo: total SMD=0.14 (−0.05, 0.34); psychosis SMD=0.17 (−0.02, 0.37); agitation SMD=0.14 (−0.05, 0.33) | 2 |

| Study type | Study | How subjects were recruited and what intervention(s) were performed[a] | Sample size[b] | How long subjects were followed | Outcome measures and main results | Rating of quality of evidence |
|---|---|---|---|---|---|---|
| 1A | Schneider et al. 2006; Sultzer et al. 2008 | Subjects with Alzheimer's disease or probable Alzheimer's disease (MMSE scores 5–26), ambulatory and residing at home or in assisted living, with moderate or greater levels of psychosis, aggression, or agitation<br>*Interventions:* placebo vs. masked, flexibly dosed olanzapine (mean dose: 5.5 mg/day), quetiapine (mean dose: 56.5 mg/day), or risperidone (mean dose: 1.0 mg/day)<br>Stable doses of cholinesterase inhibitor were permitted.<br>*Design:* multicenter, federally funded CATIE-AD trial—Phase 1 | 421 subjects randomly assigned to treatment group, with 142 receiving placebo, 100 receiving olanzapine, 94 receiving quetiapine, and 85 receiving risperidone | Median duration on Phase 1 treatment was 7.1 weeks; clinical outcomes assessed for those continuing to take antipsychotic at 12 weeks | Olanzapine vs. placebo: total SMD=0.15 (−0.11, 0.40); psychosis SMD=0.07 (−0.19, 0.33); agitation SMD=0.28 (0.02, 0.53) | 1 |
| 1A | Street et al. 2000 | Subjects with possible or probable Alzheimer's disease, residing in a nursing facility, with NPI-NH score>2<br>*Interventions:* placebo vs. fixed doses of olanzapine (5, 10, or 15 mg/day)<br>*Design:* double-blind randomized controlled trial<br>Industry-sponsored multicenter trial in the United States | 206 subjects; 66%–80% of the subjects in each study arm completed the trial | 6 weeks | Olanzapine vs. placebo: total SMD=0.30 (−0.03, 0.53); psychosis SMD=0.17 (−0.17, 0.50); agitation SMD=0.39 (0.05, 0.72) | 5 |

*Note.* 1=randomized controlled trial; 2=systematic review/meta-analysis; 3=observational; A=from AHRQ review.
AHRQ=Agency for Healthcare Research and Quality; CATIE-AD=Clinical Antipsychotic Trials of Intervention Effectiveness for Alzheimer's Disease; MMSE=Mini-Mental State Exam; NPI=Neuropsychiatric Inventory; NPI-NH=Neuropsychiatric Inventory—Nursing Home; SMD=standardized mean difference.
[a]Includes additional notes that may impact quality rating.
[b]Where applicable. Note overall $N$ as well as group $n$ for control and intervention.

*Quality of the Body of Research Evidence for Olanzapine Versus Placebo in Agitation*

*Risk of bias:* **Low**—Studies are all RCTs and vary in quality from low to high quality based on their described randomization and blinding procedures and their descriptions of study dropouts.

*Consistency:* **Consistent**—Effect sizes are overlapping and have the same size. Three of the four studies show the same direction of effect, with the fourth study showing no effect.

*Directness:* **Direct**—Studies measure overall BPSD, which is directly related to the PICOTS questions.

*Precision:* **Imprecise**—Confidence intervals are relatively narrow, but the range of confidence intervals includes negative values in two of four studies.

*Applicability:* The included studies all involve individuals with dementia, with three of the studies involving nursing home or hospital patients and two of the studies involving non-institutionalized patients. The studies include subjects from around the world, including the United States, Western Europe, and Australia/New Zealand. The doses of olanzapine that were used in the studies are consistent with usual practice.

*Dose-response relationship:* **Absent**—Two studies examined different doses of olanzapine and showed opposite effects.

*Magnitude of effect:* **Weak effect**—The effect size is quite small and barely statistically significant.

*Confounding factors:* **Absent**—No known confounding factors are present that would be likely to reduce the effect of the intervention.

*Publication bias:* **Not suspected**—There is no specific evidence to suggest selection bias.

*Overall strength of evidence:* **Moderate**—The available studies of olanzapine vs. placebo are randomized trials and have good sample sizes, but the trials are of varying quality and the imprecise nature of the results and the lack of a dose-response effect reduce confidence in the findings.

TABLE A–15. **Overview of studies comparing quetiapine with placebo for treating agitation**

| Study type | Study | How subjects were recruited and what intervention(s) were performed[a] | Sample size[b] | How long subjects were followed | Outcome measures and main results | Rating of quality of evidence |
|---|---|---|---|---|---|---|
| 1A | Ballard et al. 2005 | Subjects with a diagnosis of Alzheimer's disease, residing in nursing care facilities, with clinically significant agitation. *Interventions:* placebo vs. rivastigmine (3–6 mg BID by week 12 and >8 mg/day by week 26) vs. quetiapine (25–50 mg BID by week 12 and 50 mg BID by week 26) *Design:* double-blind randomized controlled trial. Trial conducted in England. Funded by general donations to the PIs' research program and profits from prior industry-sponsored trials. | 93 subjects; 80 started treatment (25 receiving rivastigmine, 26 quetiapine, 29 placebo), and 71 tolerated the maximum protocol dose (22 receiving rivastigmine, 23 quetiapine, 26 placebo); 56 had a baseline SIB score>10, and 46 of these subjects were included in the analysis at 6-week follow-up (14 receiving rivastigmine, 14 quetiapine, 18 placebo). | 26 weeks total; primary outcome was agitation at 6 weeks | Placebo vs. quetiapine: dementia (agitation) change in CMAI SMD=0.276 (−0.25, 0.603) Rivastigmine vs. quetiapine: dementia (agitation) change in CMAI SMD= −0.051 (−0.601, 0.499) When treated with either rivastigmine or quetiapine as compared with placebo, subjects failed to show an improvement in agitation. Relative to placebo, quetiapine, but not rivastigmine, was associated with greater cognitive decline as measured by the SIB score. | 4 |

| Study type | Study | How subjects were recruited and what intervention(s) were performed[a] | Sample size[b] | How long subjects were followed | Outcome measures and main results | Rating of quality of evidence |
|---|---|---|---|---|---|---|
| 1A | Paleacu et al. 2008 | Subjects with diagnosis of Alzheimer's disease (MMSE score<24) associated with behavioral symptoms (NPI score>6 on any item) *Interventions:* placebo vs. flexibly dosed quetiapine (50–300 mg/day; median dose: 200 mg/day) *Design:* double-blind randomized trial Industry-sponsored trial conducted in Israel | 40 enrolled; 27 completed treatment | 6 weeks | Placebo vs. quetiapine: dementia (agitation) change in NPI SMD= −0.48 (−1.11, 0.15) Significant reductions occurred in NPI total scores in both groups (79% for placebo and 68.5% for quetiapine). At 6 weeks the CGI-C score had decreased significantly in the quetiapine group ($P$=0.009) but not the placebo group ($P$=0.48). MMSE, AIMS, and SAS scores and adverse events did not show significant differences between quetiapine treatment and placebo. | 3 |

**TABLE A–15.** **Overview of studies comparing quetiapine with placebo for treating agitation** *(continued)*

| Study type | Study | How subjects were recruited and what intervention(s) were performed[a] | Sample size[b] | How long subjects were followed | Outcome measures and main results | Rating of quality of evidence |
|---|---|---|---|---|---|---|
| 1A | Schneider et al. 2006; Sultzer et al. 2008 | Subjects with Alzheimer's disease or probable Alzheimer's disease (MMSE scores 5–26), ambulatory and residing at home or in assisted living, with moderate or greater levels of psychosis, aggression, or agitation *Interventions:* placebo vs. masked flexibly dosed olanzapine (mean dose: 5.5 mg/day), quetiapine (mean dose: 56.5 mg/day), or risperidone (mean dose: 1.0 mg/day) Stable doses of cholinesterase inhibitor were permitted. *Design:* multicenter, federally funded CATIE-AD trial—Phase 1 | 421 subjects randomly assigned to treatment group, with 142 receiving placebo, 100 receiving olanzapine, 94 receiving quetiapine, and 85 receiving risperidone | Median duration on Phase 1 treatment was 7.1 weeks; clinical outcomes assessed for those continuing to receive antipsychotic at 12 weeks | Quetiapine vs. placebo: total SMD = 0.15 (−0.11, 0.40); psychosis SMD = 0.16 (−0.10, 0.42); agitation SMD = 0.20 (−0.06, 0.46) | 1 |
| 1A | Tariot et al. 2006 | Subjects with DSM-IV Alzheimer's disease (MMSE score >4), residing in a nursing facility, with psychosis and BPRS score >23 *Interventions:* placebo vs. flexibly dosed haloperidol (0.5–12 mg/day; mean dose: 1.9 mg/day) or quetiapine (25–600 mg/day; mean dose: 96.9 mg/day) *Design:* randomized controlled, double-blind trial Industry-sponsored multicenter trial in the United States | 284 subjects; data for 180 analyzed | 10 weeks | Quetiapine vs. placebo: total SMD = 0.01 (−0.29, 0.30); psychosis SMD = 0.00 (−0.29, 0.30); agitation SMD = 0.24 (−0.05, 0.54) | 4 |

**TABLE A–15. Overview of studies comparing quetiapine with placebo for treating agitation *(continued)***

| Study type | Study | How subjects were recruited and what intervention(s) were performed[a] | Sample size[b] | How long subjects were followed | Outcome measures and main results | Rating of quality of evidence |
|---|---|---|---|---|---|---|
| 1A | Zhong et al. 2007 | Subjects with possible Alzheimer's disease or vascular dementia, in long-term care facility, with agitation and PANSS-EC score>13 *Interventions:* placebo vs. quetiapine 100 mg vs. quetiapine 200 mg (adjusted according to fixed titration) *Design:* double-blind, randomized trial Industry-sponsored multicenter trial in the United States | 333 subjects | 10 weeks | Quetiapine vs. placebo: total SMD=0.04(−0.21, 0.28); psychosis SMD=−0.03 (−0.27, 0.21); agitation SMD= −0.03 (−0.27, 0.21) | 2 |

*Note.* 1=randomized controlled trial; 2=systematic review/meta-analysis; 3=observational; A=from AHRQ review. AHRQ=Agency for Healthcare Research and Quality; AIMS=Abnormal Involuntary Movement Scale; BPRS=Brief Psychiatric Rating Scale; CATIE-AD=Clinical Antipsychotic Trials of /Intervention Effectiveness for Alzheimer's Disease; CGI-C=Clinical Global Impression of Change; CMAI=Cohen-Mansfield Agitation Inventory; MMSE=Mini-Mental State Exam; NPI=Neuropsychiatric Inventory; NPI-NH=Neuropsychiatric Inventory—Nursing Home; PANSS-EC=Positive and Negative Symptom Scale—Excitement Component; PI=principal investigator; SAS=Simpson-Angus Scale; SIB=Severe Impairment Battery; SMD=standardized mean difference.
[a]Includes additional notes that may impact quality rating.
[b]Where applicable. Note overall *N* as well as group *n* for control and intervention.

### Quality of the Body of Research Evidence for Quetiapine Versus Placebo in Agitation

*Risk of bias:* **Low**—Studies are all RCTs and vary in quality from low to high quality based on their described randomization and blinding procedures and their descriptions of study dropouts.

*Consistency:* **Inconsistent**—Effect sizes in the meta-analysis are overlapping, but the direction of the effect is variable.

*Directness:* **Direct**—Studies measure agitation, which is directly related to the PICOTS questions.

*Precision:* **Imprecise**—Confidence intervals are wide for several studies, and the range of confidence intervals includes negative values in all studies included in the meta-analysis.

*Applicability:* The included studies all involve individuals with dementia, including nursing home and non-institutionalized patients. Studies include subjects from the United States. The doses of quetiapine that were used in the studies are consistent with usual practice.

*Dose-response relationship:* **Absent**—The one study that assessed two fixed doses of quetiapine for agitation found no difference in response.

*Magnitude of effect:* **Weak effect**—The effect size is quite small and not statistically significant.

*Confounding factors:* **Absent**—No known confounding factors are present that would be likely to reduce the effect of the intervention.

*Publication bias:* **Not suspected**—There is no specific evidence to suggest selection bias.

*Overall strength of evidence:* **Insufficient**—The available studies of quetiapine versus placebo are randomized trials of varying quality, and three of the five studies have good sample sizes. However, the study findings are inconsistent, and several confidence intervals are wide, and so it is difficult to draw conclusions about the data.

## Risperidone

**TABLE A–16.** **Overview of studies comparing risperidone with placebo for treating agitation**

| Study type | Study | How subjects were recruited and what intervention(s) were performed[a] | Sample size[b] | How long subjects were followed | Outcome measures and main results | Rating of quality of evidence |
|---|---|---|---|---|---|---|
| 1A | Brodaty et al. 2003, 2005 | Subjects with DSM-IV diagnosis of dementia of the Alzheimer's type, vascular dementia, or mixed dementia, residing in nursing homes, with an MMSE score<24 and significant aggressive behavior<br>*Interventions:* placebo vs. flexibly dosed risperidone (up to 2 mg/day; mean dose: 0.95 mg/day)<br>*Design:* double-blind randomized trial<br>Industry-sponsored multicenter trial in Australia/New Zealand | 345 subjects | 12 weeks | Risperidone vs. placebo total SMD=0.46 (0.23, 0.69); psychosis SMD=0.36 (0.13, 0.59); agitation SMD=0.37 (0.14, 0.59) | 3 |
| 1A | Deberdt et al. 2005 | Subjects with Alzheimer's dementia, vascular dementia, or mixed dementia, in outpatient or residential settings, with NPI or NPI-NH score>5 on hallucination and delusion items<br>*Interventions:* placebo vs. flexibly dosed olanzapine (2.5–10 mg/day; mean dose: 5.2 mg/day) or risperidone (0.5–2 mg/day; mean dose: 1.0 mg/day)<br>*Design:* double-blind randomized trial<br>Industry-sponsored multicenter trial in the United States | 494 subjects, with 94 receiving placebo, 204 receiving olanzapine, and 196 receiving risperidone | 10 weeks | Risperidone vs. placebo: total SMD= −0.13 (−0.38, 0.12); psychosis SMD= −0.03 (−0.34, 0.16); agitation SMD=0.14 (−0.11, 0.39) | 2 |

| Study type | Study | How subjects were recruited and what intervention(s) were performed[a] | Sample size[b] | How long subjects were followed | Outcome measures and main results | Rating of quality of evidence |
|---|---|---|---|---|---|---|
| 1A | De Deyn et al. 1999 | Hospitalized or institutionalized subjects with MMSE score<24 and BEHAVE-AD score>7 *Interventions:* placebo vs. flexibly dosed haloperidol (0.5–4 mg/day; mean dose: 1.2 mg/day) or risperidone (0.5–4 mg/day; mean dose: 1.1 mg/day) *Design:* randomized trial Industry-sponsored multicenter trial in the United Kingdom and Europe | 344 subjects; 68 of the 115 subjects receiving risperidone, 81 of the 115 subjects receiving haloperidol, and 74 of the 114 subjects receiving placebo completed the trial | 12 weeks | Risperidone vs. placebo: total SMD=0.12 (−0.14, 0.38); agitation SMD=0.31 (0.05, 0.57) | 4 |
| 1A | Katz et al. 1999 | Subjects with DSM-IV diagnosis of dementia of the Alzheimer's type, vascular dementia, or mixed dementia, residing in a nursing home or chronic care facility, with MMSE score<24 and significant psychotic and behavioral symptoms (BEHAVE-AD score>7) *Interventions:* placebo vs. fixed doses of risperidone at 0.5, 1, or 2 mg/day *Design:* double-blind randomized controlled trial Industry-sponsored multicenter trial in the United States | 625 subjects; 70% of the subjects completed the study | 12 weeks | Risperidone vs. placebo: total SMD=0.32 (0.11, 0.53); psychosis SMD=0.20 (−0.01, 0.41); agitation SMD=0.38 (0.17, 0.60) | 4 |

| Study type | Study | How subjects were recruited and what intervention(s) were performed[a] | Sample size[b] | How long subjects were followed | Outcome measures and main results | Rating of quality of evidence |
|---|---|---|---|---|---|---|
| 1A | Mintzer et al. 2006 | Subjects who were mobile and had symptoms that met criteria for Alzheimer's dementia (MMSE scores 5–23), residing in nursing homes or long-term care, with psychosis *Interventions:* placebo vs. flexibly dosed risperidone (0.5-1.5 mg/day; mean dose: 1.03 mg/day) *Design:* randomized controlled trial Industry-sponsored multicenter trial in the United States | 473 subjects randomly assigned to treatment group, with 238 receiving placebo and 235 receiving risperidone; 354 completed the study | 8 weeks, after 1–16 days of placebo run-in/washout | Risperidone vs. placebo: total SMD= −0.01 (−0.21, 0.18); psychosis SMD=0.17 (−0.02, 0.36); agitation SMD=0.04 (−0.16, 0.23) | 3 |
| 1A | Schneider et al. 2006; Sultzer et al. 2008 | Subjects with Alzheimer's disease or probable Alzheimer's disease (MMSE scores 5–26), ambulatory and residing at home or in assisted living, with moderate or greater levels of psychosis, aggression, or agitation *Interventions:* placebo vs. masked, flexibly dosed olanzapine (mean dose: 5.5 mg/day), quetiapine (mean dose: 56.5 mg/day), or risperidone (mean dose: 1.0 mg/day) Stable doses of cholinesterase inhibitor were permitted. *Design:* multicenter, federally funded CATIE-AD trial—Phase 1 | 421 subjects randomly assigned to treatment group, with 142 receiving placebo, 100 receiving olanzapine, 94 receiving quetiapine, and 85 receiving risperidone | Median duration on Phase 1 treatment was 7.1 weeks; clinical outcomes assessed for those continuing to take antipsychotic at 12 weeks | Risperidone vs. placebo: total SMD=0.40 (0.13, 0.68); psychosis SMD=0.38 (0.11, 0.66); agitation SMD=0.10 (−0.17, 0.37) | 1 |

*Note.* 1=randomized controlled trial; 2=systematic review/meta-analysis; 3=observational; A=from AHRQ review.
AHRQ=Agency for Healthcare Research and Quality; BEHAVE-AD=Behavioral Pathology in Alzheimer's Disease; CATIE-AD = Clinical Antipsychotic Trials of Intervention Effectiveness for Alzheimer's Disease; MMSE=Mini-Mental State Exam; NPI=Neuropsychiatric Inventory; NPI-NH=Neuropsychiatric Inventory—Nursing Home; SMD=standardized mean difference.
[a]Includes additional notes that may impact quality rating.
[b]Where applicable. Note overall *N* as well as group *n* for control and intervention.

*Quality of the Body of Research Evidence for Risperidone Versus Placebo in Agitation*

*Risk of bias:* **Low**—Studies are all RCTs and vary in quality from low to high quality based on their described randomization and blinding procedures and their descriptions of study dropouts.

*Consistency:* **Consistent**—Effect sizes are overlapping, and the direction of the effect favors risperidone in all of the studies.

*Directness:* **Direct**—Studies measure agitation, which is directly related to the PICOTS questions.

*Precision:* **Imprecise**—The confidence intervals are narrow, but the range of confidence intervals includes negative values for three of the studies.

*Applicability:* The included studies all involve individuals with dementia, including nursing home or hospital patients and non-institutionalized patients. Studies include subjects from around the world, including the United States, United Kingdom, Western Europe, and Australia/New Zealand. The doses of risperidone that were used in the studies are consistent with usual practice.

*Dose-response relationship:* **Absent**—One study examined different fixed doses of risperidone, and confidence intervals suggest a dose-response effect in the treatment of agitation, but these dose-response relationships did not reach statistical significance.

*Magnitude of effect:* **Weak effect**—The effect size is small but statistically significant.

*Confounding factors:* **Absent**—No known confounding factors are present that would be likely to reduce the effect of the intervention.

*Publication bias:* **Not suspected**—There is no specific evidence to suggest selection bias.

*Overall strength of evidence:* **Moderate**—The available studies of risperidone versus placebo are randomized trials of varying quality with good sample sizes. The overall effect size according to the AHRQ meta-analysis is small and there is some imprecision; however, the directions of the findings are consistent.

## Quality of the Body of Research Evidence for Second-Generation Antipsychotics Versus Placebo in Agitation

*Risk of bias:* **Low**—Studies are all RCTs, and the vast majority are double-blind trials. They vary in quality from low to high quality based on their described randomization and blinding procedures and their descriptions of study dropouts.

*Consistency:* **Consistent**—Effect sizes are generally overlapping, and the majority of the studies show an effect in the direction of SGA benefit. The AHRQ meta-analysis shows small but statistically significant effects for olanzapine and risperidone on agitation.

*Directness:* **Direct**—Studies measure agitation, which is directly related to the PICOTS questions.

*Precision:* **Imprecise**—Confidence intervals for individual studies are relatively narrow, with the exception of two studies of quetiapine, but the range of confidence intervals includes negative values in over half of the studies.

*Applicability:* The included studies all involve individuals with dementia, including nursing home or hospital patients and non-institutionalized patients. The studies include subjects from around the world, including the United States, Canada, Western Europe, and Australia/New Zealand. The doses of SGA medications that were used in the studies are consistent with usual practice.

*Dose-response relationship:* **Absent**—For aripiprazole, quetiapine, and risperidone, only one study of each medication is available that assesses differing doses; two studies are available for olanzapine, with no consistency in results. There appears to be a trend for dose-response relationships for risperidone based on the confidence intervals, but these dose-response relationships did not show statistical differences.

*Magnitude of effect:* **Weak effect**—The effect sizes are small for all medications.

*Confounding factors:* **Absent**—No known confounding factors are present that would be likely to reduce the effect of the intervention.

*Publication bias:* **Not suspected**—There is no specific evidence to suggest selection bias.

*Overall strength of evidence:* **Moderate**—A significant number of randomized trials of SGAs versus placebo are available. Trials are of varying quality, but most have good sample sizes. The majority of the studies show a beneficial effect, albeit a small one, for treatment with the antipsychotic as compared with placebo.

# Second-Generation Antipsychotic Versus Haloperidol

## Overview and Quality of Individual Studies

**TABLE A–17.** Overview of studies comparing second-generation antipsychotics with haloperidol for treating agitation

| Study type | Study | How subjects were recruited and what intervention(s) were performed[a] | Sample size[b] | How long subjects were followed | Outcome measures and main results | Rating of quality of evidence |
|---|---|---|---|---|---|---|
| 1 | Chan et al. 2001 | Inpatients or outpatients with a DSM-IV diagnosis of dementia of Alzheimer's type or vascular dementia associated with behavioral symptoms. *Interventions:* flexibly dosed haloperidol (0.5–2 mg/day; mean dose: 0.90 mg/day) vs. risperidone (0.5–2 mg/day; mean dose: 0.85 mg/day) *Design:* double-blind randomized controlled trial. Industry-sponsored multicenter trial in Hong Kong | 58 subjects | 3 months | Haloperidol vs. risperidone: change in BEHAVE-AD dementia (aggressiveness) SMD=0.057 (−0.472, 0.585); change in BEHAVE-AD dementia (psychosis) SMD=−0.383 (−0.917, 0.15) Scores on the CMAI and BEHAVE-AD were significantly improved by both haloperidol and risperidone, with no significant differences between the two treatments. Haloperidol-treated patients, but not risperidone-treated patients, showed an increase in EPS on the SAS. | 3 |
| 1A | De Deyn et al. 1999 | Hospitalized or institutionalized subjects with MMSE score<24 and a BEHAVE-AD score>7 *Interventions:* placebo vs. flexibly dosed haloperidol (0.5–4 mg/day; mean dose: 1.2 mg/day) or risperidone (0.5–4 mg/day; mean dose: 1.1 mg/day) *Design:* randomized trial. Industry-sponsored multicenter trial in the United Kingdom and Europe | 344 subjects | 12 weeks | Risperidone vs. haloperidol: total SMD= −0.19 (−0.45, 0.07); agitation SMD=−0.07 (−0.19, 0.33) | 4 |

| Study type | Study | How subjects were recruited and what intervention(s) were performed[a] | Sample size[b] | How long subjects were followed | Outcome measures and main results | Rating of quality of evidence |
|---|---|---|---|---|---|---|
| 1A | Savaskan et al. 2006 | Inpatients with ICD-10 Alzheimer's disease and associated behavioral symptoms<br>*Interventions:* haloperidol (0.5–4 mg/day; mean dose: 1.9 mg/day) vs. quetiapine (25–200 mg/day; mean dose: 125 mg/day); fixed titration schedule with weekly dose increments to final dose<br>*Design:* open-label randomized controlled trial<br>Trial conducted in Switzerland; two of the three investigators were noted to be supported by an industry-sponsored grant. | 30 subjects enrolled; 4 dropped out, and 4 had missing data; data for 22 analyzed | 5 weeks, after run-in period of up to 7 days | Quetiapine vs. haloperidol: total SMD=0.99 (0.10, 1.88); agitation SMD=0.06 (−0.78, 0.89) | 2 |
| 1 | Suh et al. 2004, 2006 | Subjects residing in a nursing facility with a diagnosis of Alzheimer's disease, vascular dementia, or mixed dementia associated with behavioral disturbance (FAST score>3, BEHAVE-D score>7, CMAI score>2 on at least two items)<br>*Interventions:* flexibly dosed risperidone (0.5–1.5 mg/day; mean dose: 0.80 mg/day) vs. haloperidol (0.5-1.5 mg/day; mean dose: 0.83 mg/day)<br>*Design:* double-blind, crossover, randomized trial<br>Industry-sponsored trial at a single center in Korea | 120 subjects | 18 weeks | Compared with haloperidol treatment, risperidone treatment was associated with greater clinical improvement on total and subscale scores of the Korean version of BEHAVE-AD, on total and subscale scores of the Korean version of CMAI, and on the CGI-C, as well as a lower frequency of EPS. | 4 |
| 1A | Tariot et al. 2006 | Subjects with DSM-IV Alzheimer's disease (MMSE score>4), residing in a nursing facility, with psychosis and BPRS score>23<br>*Interventions:* placebo vs. flexibly dosed haloperidol (0.5–12 mg/day; mean dose: 1.9 mg/day) or quetiapine (25–600 mg/day; mean dose: 96.9 mg/day)<br>*Design:* double-blind randomized controlled trial<br>Industry-sponsored multicenter trial in the United States | 284 subjects; data for 180 analyzed | 10 weeks | Quetiapine vs. haloperidol: total SMD=0.16 (−0.16, 0.47); agitation SMD= 0.04 (−0.26, 0.34) | 4 |

**TABLE A–17. Overview of studies comparing second-generation antipsychotics with haloperidol for treating agitation (continued)**

| Study type | Study | How subjects were recruited and what intervention(s) were performed[a] | Sample size[b] | How long subjects were followed | Outcome measures and main results | Rating of quality of evidence |
|---|---|---|---|---|---|---|
| 1A | Verhey et al. 2006 | Subjects with DSM-IV diagnosis of dementia, living in nursing homes or their own homes, who were judged to be in need of treatment for clinically significant agitation (CMAI score >44) *Interventions:* haloperidol (1–3 mg/day; mean dose: 1.75 mg) vs. olanzapine (2.5–7.5 mg/day; mean dose: 4.71 mg) *Design:* double-blind, two-arm randomized controlled study Randomization took place after a 3- to 11-day washout. Multicenter trial conducted in the Netherlands; funding source not noted | 59 subjects; 1 excluded for missing data; 3 patients, all of whom were in the olanzapine group, withdrew from the study | 5 weeks total; titration for up to 2 weeks, and at least 3 weeks at stable dose | Olanzapine vs. haloperidol: total SMD= −0.18 (−0.77, 0.41); agitation SMD=−0.21 (−0.73, 0.31) AHRQ does not report SMD for psychosis comparison, but the change in the NPI psychosis item showed no significant difference in the scores for the two treatments. | 3 |

*Note.* 1=randomized controlled trial; 2=systematic review/meta-analysis; 3=observational; A=from AHRQ review. AHRQ=Agency for Healthcare Research and Quality; BEHAVE-AD=Behavioral Pathology in Alzheimer's Disease; BPRS=Brief Psychiatric Rating Scale; CATIE-AD=Clinical Antipsychotic Trials of Intervention Effectiveness for Alzheimer's Disease; CGI-C=Clinical Global Impression of Change; CMAI= Cohen-Mansfield Agitation Inventory; EPS=extrapyramidal side effects; FAST=Functional Assessment Staging; MMSE=Mini-Mental State Exam; NPI=Neuropsychiatric Inventory; SAS=Simpson-Angus Scale; SMD=standardized mean difference.
[a]Includes additional notes that may impact quality rating.
[b]Where applicable. Note overall *N* as well as group *n* for control and intervention.

## Quality of the Body of Research Evidence for Second-Generation Antipsychotics Versus Haloperidol in Agitation

*Risk of bias:* **Low**—Studies are all randomized trials with one crossover trial. The studies are of moderate to high quality based on their described randomization and blinding procedures and their descriptions of study dropouts.

*Consistency:* **Consistent**—Effect sizes are consistent in showing minimal difference between haloperidol and the comparison SGAs.

*Directness:* **Direct**—Studies measure agitation, which is directly related to the PICOTS questions.

*Precision:* **Imprecise**—Confidence intervals are variable in width, and several confidence intervals are extremely wide.

*Applicability:* The included studies all involve individuals with dementia, with the majority of the studies including nursing home or hospital patients. Studies include subjects from around the world, including the United States, United Kingdom, Western Europe, Hong Kong, and Japan. The doses of antipsychotic that were used in the studies are consistent with usual practice.

*Dose-response relationship:* **Not applicable for this comparison.**

*Magnitude of effect:* **Not applicable.**

*Confounding factors:* **Absent**—No known confounding factors are present that would be likely to reduce the effect of the intervention.

*Publication bias:* **Not suspected**—There is no specific evidence to suggest selection bias.

*Overall strength of evidence:* **Low**—The available studies of SGA medications as compared with haloperidol that assessed agitation include five randomized parallel-arm trials and one randomized crossover trial. The trials are of varying quality, and some have small sample sizes. For the trials that were included in the AHRQ meta-analysis, the effect size is small and does not show evidence of a difference between haloperidol and SGAs overall. Studies that were not a part of the AHRQ analysis are consistent with this observation. For individual agents, there are no more than two studies for each drug, and several of the studies have extremely wide confidence intervals.

## Olanzapine or Quetiapine Versus Risperidone

### Overview and Quality of Individual Studies

**TABLE A–18. Overview of studies comparing olanzapine or quetiapine with risperidone for treating agitation**

| Study type | Study | How subjects were recruited and what intervention(s) were performed[a] | Sample size[b] | How long subjects were followed | Outcome measures and main results | Rating of quality of evidence |
|---|---|---|---|---|---|---|
| 1A | Deberdt et al. 2005 | Subjects with Alzheimer's dementia, vascular dementia, or mixed dementia and NPI or NPI-NH score >5 on hallucination and delusion items<br>*Interventions:* placebo vs. flexibly dosed olanzapine (2.5–10 mg/day; mean dose: 5.2 mg/day) or risperidone (0.5–2 mg/day; mean dose: 1.0 mg/day)<br>*Design:* double-blind randomized trial<br>Industry-sponsored multicenter trial in the United States | 494 subjects, with 94 receiving placebo, 204 receiving olanzapine, and 196 receiving risperidone | 10 weeks | Olanzapine vs. risperidone: total SMD=0.10 (−0.10, 0.30); psychosis SMD=−0.03 (−0.23, 0.17); agitation SMD= −0.04 (−0.24, 0.16) | 2 |
| 1A | Schneider et al. 2006; Sultzer et al. 2008 | Subjects with Alzheimer's disease or probable Alzheimer's disease (MMSE scores 5–26), ambulatory and residing at home or in assisted living facilities, with moderate or greater levels of psychosis, aggression, or agitation<br>*Interventions:* placebo vs. masked, flexibly dosed olanzapine (mean dose: 5.5 mg/day), quetiapine (mean dose: 56.5 mg/day), or risperidone (mean dose: 1.0 mg/day)<br>Stable doses of cholinesterase inhibitor were permitted.<br>*Design:* multicenter, federally funded CATIE-AD trial— Phase 1 | 421 subjects randomly assigned to treatment group, with 142 receiving placebo, 100 receiving olanzapine, 94 receiving quetiapine, and 85 receiving risperidone | Median duration on Phase 1 treatment was 7.1 weeks; clinical outcomes assessed for those continuing to take antipsychotic at 12 weeks | Olanzapine vs. risperidone: total SMD=−0.27 (−0.56, 0.02); psychosis SMD= −0.27 (−0.56, 0.02); agitation SMD= 0.17 (−0.12, 0.16) Quetiapine vs. risperidone: total SMD=−0.24 (−0.53, 0.06); psychosis SMD= −0.24 (−0.54, 0.05); agitation SMD= 0.10 (−0.20, 0.39) | 1 |

**TABLE A–18.** Overview of studies comparing olanzapine or quetiapine with risperidone for treating agitation *(continued)*

| Study type | Study | How subjects were recruited and what intervention(s) were performed[a] | Sample size[b] | How long subjects were followed | Outcome measures and main results | Rating of quality of evidence |
|---|---|---|---|---|---|---|
| 1A | Rainer et al. 2007 | Outpatients with mild to moderate dementia of the Alzheimer's, vascular, mixed, or frontotemporal lobe type according to DSM-IV and ICD-10 who had behavioral disturbance and NPI subitem scores relating to psychosis or agitation/aggression *Interventions:* flexibly dosed quetiapine (50–400 mg/day; mean dose: 77 mg/day) vs. risperidone (0.5–4 mg/day; mean dose: 0.9 mg/day) *Design:* single-blind, parallel-group randomized trial Investigator-sponsored multi-center trial in Western Europe | 72 subjects, with 65 subjects in the ITT population; 34 receiving quetiapine and 31 receiving risperidone | 8 weeks | Quetiapine vs. risperidone: total SMD=−0.06 (−0.55, 0.43); agitation SMD=−0.17 (−0.66, 0.32) | 3 |

*Note.* 1=randomized controlled trial; 2=systematic review/meta-analysis; 3=observational; A=from AHRQ review. AHRQ=Agency for Healthcare Research and Quality; CATIE-AD=Clinical Antipsychotic Trials of Intervention Effectiveness for Alzheimer's Disease; ITT=intention to treat; MMSE=Mini-Mental State Exam; NPI=Neuropsychiatric Inventory; NPI-NH=Neuropsychiatric Inventory—Nursing Home; SMD=standardized mean difference.
[a]Includes additional notes that may impact quality rating.
[b]Where applicable. Note overall *N* as well as group *n* for control and intervention.

## Quality of the Body of Research Evidence for Olanzapine or Quetiapine Versus Risperidone in Agitation

*Risk of bias:* **Moderate**—Studies are all RCTs but vary in quality from low to moderate based on their described randomization and blinding procedures and their descriptions of study dropouts.

*Consistency:* **Inconsistent**—Effect sizes are overlapping and show no prominent differences between risperidone and either olanzapine or quetiapine in the limited number of studies available. However, the direction of the effect is variable.

*Directness:* **Direct**—Studies measure agitation, which is directly related to the PICOTS questions.

*Precision:* **Imprecise**—Confidence intervals are relatively wide, and the range of confidence intervals includes negative values in all four studies.

*Applicability:* The included studies all involve individuals with dementia, including patients in institutional and outpatient settings. The studies include subjects from around the world, including the United States and Western Europe. The doses of medication that were used in the studies are consistent with usual practice.

*Dose-response relationship:* **Not applicable to this comparison**.

*Magnitude of effect:* **Not applicable**.

*Confounding factors:* **Absent**—No known confounding factors are present that would be likely to reduce the effect of the intervention.

*Publication bias:* **Not suspected**—There is no specific evidence to suggest selection bias.

*Overall strength of evidence:* **Low**—The available studies of risperidone as compared with olanzapine or quetiapine are randomized trials of low to moderate quality. The studies vary in their sample sizes. In addition, several of the confidence intervals are wide. However, they are consistent in showing no significant differences between risperidone and either olanzapine or quetiapine.

## 1C. Efficacy and Comparative Effectiveness of Second-Generation Antipsychotics for Treatment of Psychosis

### Second-Generation Antipsychotic Versus Placebo

#### Overview and Quality of Individual Studies

Aripiprazole

**TABLE A–19.** Overview of studies comparing aripiprazole with placebo for treating psychosis

| Study type | Study | How subjects were recruited and what intervention(s) were performed[a] | Sample size[b] | How long subjects were followed | Outcome measures and main results | Rating of quality of evidence |
|---|---|---|---|---|---|---|
| 1A | Breder et al. 2004; Mintzer et al. 2007 | Nursing home residents with MMSE scores 6–22 and NPI or NPI-NH score>5 for hallucinations and delusions *Interventions:* placebo vs. three fixed doses of aripiprazole (2 mg, 5 mg, 10 mg) *Design:* double-blind randomized controlled trial Industry-sponsored multicenter trial conducted in long-term care facilities internationally, including the United States and Canada | 487 subjects enrolled; data for 284 analyzed | 10 weeks | Aripiprazole vs. placebo: total SMD=0.16 (−0.05, 0.37); psychosis SMD=0.24 (0.03, 0.45); agitation SMD=0.31 (0.10, 0.52) | 1, 2 |
| 1A | De Deyn et al. 2005 | Non-institutionalized subjects with Alzheimer's disease and psychosis *Interventions:* placebo vs. aripiprazole (2–15 mg/day) *Design:* double-blind randomized controlled trials Industry-sponsored multicenter trial conducted in the United States, Canada, Western Europe, and Australia/New Zealand | 208 subjects | 10 weeks | Aripiprazole vs. placebo: total SMD=0.06 (−0.21, 0.34); psychosis SMD=0.16 (−0.12, 0.43) | 3 |

**TABLE A–19.** Overview of studies comparing aripiprazole with placebo for treating psychosis *(continued)*

| Study type | Study | How subjects were recruited and what intervention(s) were performed[a] | Sample size[b] | How long subjects were followed | Outcome measures and main results | Rating of quality of evidence |
|---|---|---|---|---|---|---|
| 1A | Streim et al. 2008 | Nursing home residents with Alzheimer's disease and psychosis<br>*Interventions:* placebo vs. aripiprazole (0.7–15 mg/day; average dose: 8.6 mg/day)<br>*Design:* double-blind randomized controlled trial<br>Industry-sponsored multicenter trial conducted in long-term care facilities in the United States | 256 subjects enrolled; data for 151 analyzed | 10 weeks, after 1-week washout | Aripiprazole vs. placebo: total SMD=0.36 (0.11, 0.61); psychosis SMD=−0.02 (−0.27, 0.23); agitation SMD= 0.30 (0.05, 0.55) | 2 |

*Note.* 1=randomized controlled trial; 2=systematic review/meta-analysis; 3=observational; A=from AHRQ review. AHRQ=Agency for Healthcare Research and Quality; MMSE=Mini-Mental State Exam; NPI=Neuropsychiatric Inventory; NPI-NH = Neuropsychiatric Inventory—Nursing Home; SMD=standardized mean difference.
[a]Includes additional notes that may impact quality rating.
[b]Where applicable. Note overall *N* as well as group *n* for control and intervention.

### Quality of the Body of Research Evidence for Aripiprazole Versus Placebo in Psychotic Symptoms

*Risk of bias:* **Low**—Studies are all RCTs and are of low to moderate quality based on their described randomization and blinding procedures and their descriptions of study dropouts.

*Consistency:* **Consistent**—Effect sizes are overlapping and have the same size. Two of the three studies have the same direction of effect, and the third study shows no effect.

*Directness:* **Direct**—Studies measure psychosis, which is directly related to the PICOTS questions.

*Precision:* **Imprecise**—Confidence intervals are relatively narrow, but the range of confidence intervals includes negative values in two of the three studies.

*Applicability:* The included studies all involve individuals with dementia, with two of the studies in nursing home or hospital patients and one study in non-institutionalized patients. The studies include subjects from around the world, including the United States, Canada, Western Europe, and Australia/New Zealand. The doses of aripiprazole that were used in the studies are consistent with usual practice.

*Dose-response relationship:* **Absent**—A single study examined the effect of different doses of aripiprazole relative to placebo, and inspection of confidence intervals appears to show a dose-response effect between 2 mg and 10 mg; however, this did not show statistical significance.

*Magnitude of effect:* **Weak effect**—The effect size is small and not statistically significant.

*Confounding factors:* **Absent**—No known confounding factors are present that would be likely to reduce the effect of the intervention.

*Publication bias:* **Not suspected**—There is no specific evidence to suggest selection bias.

*Overall strength of evidence:* **Low**—The three available studies of aripiprazole vs. placebo are randomized trials of low to moderate quality and have good sample sizes. However, there was a lack of consistency in study conclusions.

## Olanzapine

**TABLE A–20. Overview of studies comparing olanzapine with placebo for treating psychosis**

| Study type | Study | How subjects were recruited and what intervention(s) were performed[a] | Sample size[b] | How long subjects were followed | Outcome measures and main results | Rating of quality of evidence |
|---|---|---|---|---|---|---|
| 1A | Deberdt et al. 2005 | Subjects with Alzheimer's dementia, vascular dementia, or mixed dementia, in outpatient or residential settings, with NPI or NPI-NH>5 on hallucination and delusion items<br>*Interventions:* placebo vs. flexibly dosed olanzapine (2.5–10 mg/day; mean dose: 5.2 mg/day) or risperidone (0.5–2 mg/day; mean dose: 1.0 mg/day)<br>*Design:* double-blind randomized trial<br>Industry-sponsored multicenter trial in the United States | 494 subjects, with 94 receiving placebo, 204 receiving olanzapine, and 196 receiving risperidone | 10 weeks | Olanzapine vs. placebo: total SMD = −0.02 (−0.27, 0.23); psychosis SMD = −0.12 (−0.36, 0.13); agitation SMD = 0.09 (−0.16, 0.34) | 2 |
| 1A | De Deyn et al. 2004 | Subjects with Alzheimer's disease (MMSE scores 5–26), in long-term care settings, with hallucinations or delusions<br>*Interventions:* placebo vs. fixed-dose olanzapine (1, 2.5, 5, or 7.5 mg/day)<br>*Design:* double-blind randomized trial<br>Industry–sponsored multicenter trial in Europe, Israel, Lebanon, Australia/New Zealand, and South Africa | 652 subjects; 65%–75% of the subjects in each study arm completed the trial | 10 weeks | Olanzapine vs. placebo: total SMD = 0.14 (−0.05, 0.34); psychosis SMD = 0.17 (−0.02, 0.37); agitation SMD = 0.14 (−0.05, 0.33) | 2 |

**TABLE A-20. Overview of studies comparing olanzapine with placebo for treating psychosis** *(continued)*

| Study type | Study | How subjects were recruited and what intervention(s) were performed[a] | Sample size[b] | How long subjects were followed | Outcome measures and main results | Rating of quality of evidence |
|---|---|---|---|---|---|---|
| 1A | Schneider et al. 2006; Sultzer et al. 2008 | Subjects with Alzheimer's disease or probable Alzheimer's disease (MMSE scores 5–26), ambulatory and residing at home or in assisted living facilities, with moderate or greater levels of psychosis, aggression, or agitation *Interventions:* placebo vs. masked, flexibly dosed olanzapine (mean dose: 5.5 mg/day), quetiapine (mean dose: 56.5 mg/day), or risperidone (mean dose: 1.0 mg/day) Stable doses of cholinesterase inhibitor were permitted. *Design:* multicenter, federally funded CATIE-AD trial—Phase 1 | 421 subjects randomly assigned to treatment group, with 142 receiving placebo, 100 receiving olanzapine, 94 receiving quetiapine, and 85 receiving risperidone | Median duration on Phase 1 treatment was 7.1 weeks; clinical outcomes assessed for those continuing to take antipsychotic at 12 weeks | Olanzapine vs. placebo: total SMD=0.15 (−0.11, 0.40); psychosis SMD=0.07 (−0.19, 0.33); agitation SMD=0.28 (0.02, 0.53) | 1 |
| 1A | Street et al. 2000 | Subjects with possible or probable Alzheimer's disease, resided in a nursing facility, with NPI-NH score>2 *Interventions:* placebo vs. fixed doses of olanzapine (5, 10, or 15 mg/day) *Design:* double-blind randomized controlled trial Industry-sponsored multicenter trial in the United States | 206 subjects; 66%–80% of individuals in each study arm completed the trial | 6 weeks | Olanzapine vs. placebo: total SMD=0.30 (−0.03, 0.53); psychosis SMD=0.17 (−0.17, 0.50); agitation SMD=0.39 (0.05, 0.72) | 5 |

*Note.* 1=randomized controlled trial; 2=systematic review/meta-analysis; 3=observational; A=from AHRQ review. AHRQ=Agency for Healthcare Research and Quality; CATIE-AD=Clinical Antipsychotic Trials of Intervention Effectiveness for Alzheimer's Disease; MMSE=Mini-Mental State Exam; NPI=Neuropsychiatric Inventory; NPI-NH=Neuropsychiatric Inventory—Nursing Home; SMD=standardized mean difference.
[a]Includes additional notes that may impact quality rating.
[b]Where applicable. Note overall *N* as well as group *n* for control and intervention.

*Quality of the Body of Research Evidence for Olanzapine Versus Placebo in Psychotic Symptoms*

*Risk of bias:* **Low**—Studies are all RCTs and vary in quality from low to high quality based on their described randomization and blinding procedures and their descriptions of study dropouts.

*Consistency:* **Inconsistent**—Effect sizes are overlapping, and some are wide. Three of the four studies show the same direction of effect, with the fourth study showing the opposite effect. In none of the studies is the effect statistically significant.

*Directness:* **Direct**—Studies measure psychosis, which is directly related to the PICOTS questions.

*Practice Guideline on Use of Antipsychotics to Treat Agitation or Psychosis in Patients With Dementia* **103**

*Precision:* **Imprecise**—Confidence intervals are relatively wide, and the range of confidence intervals includes negative values in all five studies.

*Applicability:* The included studies all involve individuals with dementia, including nursing home or hospital patients and non-institutionalized patients. However, in one of the studies, patients were specifically excluded if they had psychotic symptoms at baseline. The studies include subjects from around the world, including the United States, Western Europe, and Australia/New Zealand. The doses of olanzapine that were used in the studies are consistent with usual practice.

*Dose-response relationship:* **Absent**—Two studies examined different doses of olanzapine and showed varying effects with olanzapine dose with no consistent trends or statistically significant differences based on dose.

*Magnitude of effect:* **Weak effect**—The effect size is quite small and not statistically significant.

*Confounding factors:* **Absent**—No known confounding factors are present that would be likely to reduce the effect of the intervention.

*Publication bias:* **Not suspected**—There is no specific evidence to suggest selection bias.

*Overall strength of evidence:* **Insufficient**—The available studies of olanzapine vs. placebo are randomized trials of varying quality and have good sample sizes. However, the effect size of these trials is small according to the AHRQ meta-analysis, the confidence intervals are relatively wide, and the findings are inconsistent, and so it is difficult to draw conclusions with any degree of confidence.

# Quetiapine

**TABLE A–21. Overview of studies comparing quetiapine with placebo for treating psychosis**

| Study type | Study | How subjects were recruited and what intervention(s) were performed[a] | Sample size[b] | How long subjects were followed | Outcome measures and main results | Rating of quality of evidence |
|---|---|---|---|---|---|---|
| 1A | Schneider et al. 2006; Sultzer et al. 2008 | Subjects with Alzheimer's disease or probable Alzheimer's disease (MMSE scores 5–26), ambulatory and residing at home or in assisted living facilities, with moderate or greater levels of psychosis, aggression, or agitation<br>*Interventions:* placebo vs. masked, flexibly dosed olanzapine (mean dose: 5.5 mg/day), quetiapine (mean dose: 56.5 mg/day), or risperidone (mean dose: 1.0 mg/day)<br>Stable doses of cholinesterase inhibitor were permitted.<br>*Design:* multicenter, federally funded CATIE-AD trial—Phase 1 | 421 subjects randomly assigned to treatment group, with 142 receiving placebo, 100 receiving olanzapine, 94 receiving quetiapine, and 85 receiving risperidone | Median duration on Phase 1 treatment was 7.1 weeks; clinical outcomes assessed for those continuing to take antipsychotic at 12 weeks | Quetiapine vs. placebo: total SMD = 0.15 (−0.11, 0.40); psychosis SMD = 0.16 (−0.10, 0.42); agitation SMD = 0.10 (−0.17, 0.37) | 1 |
| 1A | Tariot et al. 2006 | Subjects with DSM-IV Alzheimer's disease (MMSE score > 4), residing in a nursing facility, with psychosis and BPRS score > 23<br>*Interventions:* placebo vs. flexibly dosed haloperidol (0.5–12 mg/day; mean dose: 1.9 mg/day) or quetiapine (25–600 mg/day; mean dose: 96.9 mg/day)<br>*Design:* double-blind randomized controlled trial<br>Industry-sponsored multicenter trial in the United States | 284 subjects; data for 180 analyzed | 10 weeks | Quetiapine vs. placebo: total SMD = 0.01 (−0.29, 0.30); psychosis SMD = 0.00 (−0.29, 0.30); agitation SMD = 0.25 (−0.05, 0.54) | 4 |

**TABLE A–21.** Overview of studies comparing quetiapine with placebo for treating psychosis *(continued)*

| Study type | Study | How subjects were recruited and what intervention(s) were performed[a] | Sample size[b] | How long subjects were followed | Outcome measures and main results | Rating of quality of evidence |
|---|---|---|---|---|---|---|
| 1A | Zhong et al. 2007 | Subjects with possible Alzheimer's disease or vascular dementia, in long-term care facility, with agitation and PANSS-EC score>13 *Interventions:* placebo vs. quetiapine 100 mg vs. quetiapine 200 mg (dose adjusted according to fixed titration) *Design:* double-blind randomized trial Industry-sponsored multicenter trial in the United States | 333 subjects | 10 weeks | Quetiapine vs. placebo: total SMD= 0.04 (−0.21, 0.28); psychosis SMD= −0.03 (−0.27, 0.21); agitation SMD= −0.03 (−0.27, 0.21) | 2 |

*Note.* 1=randomized controlled trial; 2=systematic review/meta-analysis; 3=observational; A=from AHRQ review. AHRQ=Agency for Healthcare Research and Quality; BPRS=Brief Psychiatric Rating Scale; CATIE-AD=Clinical Antipsychotic Trials of Intervention Effectiveness for Alzheimer's Disease; MMSE=Mini-Mental State Exam; PANSS-EC=Positive and Negative Symptom Scale—Excitement Component; SMD = standardized mean difference.
[a]Includes additional notes that may impact quality rating.
[b]Where applicable. Note overall $N$ as well as group $n$ for control and intervention.

### Quality of the Body of Research Evidence for Quetiapine Versus Placebo in Psychotic Symptoms

*Risk of bias:* **Low**—Studies are all RCTs and vary in quality from low to high quality based on their described randomization and blinding procedures and their descriptions of study dropouts.

*Consistency:* **Inconsistent**—Effect sizes in the meta-analysis are overlapping and have the same magnitude. The three studies in the meta-analysis have varying directions of effect, and in none of the studies is the effect statistically significant.

*Directness:* **Direct**—Studies measure psychosis, which is directly related to the PICOTS questions.

*Precision:* **Imprecise**—Confidence intervals are narrow, but the range of confidence intervals includes negative values in all studies included in the meta-analysis.

*Applicability:* The included studies all involve individuals with dementia, with two of the studies including nursing home or hospital patients and one study including non-institutionalized patients. Studies include subjects from the United States. The doses of quetiapine that were used in the studies are consistent with usual practice.

*Dose-response relationship:* **Absent**—One study examined different doses of quetiapine and showed a difference in effect based on dose.

*Magnitude of effect:* **Weak effect**—The effect size is quite small and not statistically significant.

*Confounding factors:* **Absent**—No known confounding factors are present that would be likely to reduce the effect of the intervention.

*Publication bias:* **Not suspected**—There is no specific evidence to suggest selection bias.

*Overall strength of evidence:* **Insufficient**—The available studies of quetiapine versus placebo are randomized trials with good sample sizes. They are of varying quality, and the direction of findings in the studies is variable, and so it is difficult to draw conclusions with any degree of confidence. None of the studies included in the meta-analysis showed a statistically significant benefit.

## Risperidone

**TABLE A–22. Overview of studies comparing risperidone with placebo for treating psychosis**

| Study type | Study | How subjects were recruited and what intervention(s) were performed[a] | Sample size[b] | How long subjects were followed | Outcome measures and main results | Rating of quality of evidence |
|---|---|---|---|---|---|---|
| 1A | Brodaty et al. 2003, 2005 | Subjects with a DSM-IV diagnosis of dementia of the Alzheimer's type, vascular dementia, or mixed dementia, residing in nursing homes, with MMSE score<24 and significant aggressive behavior<br>*Interventions:* placebo vs. flexibly dosed risperidone (up to 2 mg/day; mean dose: 0.95 mg/day)<br>*Design:* double-blind randomized trial<br>Industry-sponsored multicenter trial in Australia/New Zealand | 345 subjects | 12 weeks | Risperidone vs. placebo: total SMD=0.46 (0.23, 0.69); psychosis SMD=0.36 (0.13, 0.59); agitation SMD=0.37 (0.14, 0.59) | 3 |
| 1A | Deberdt et al. 2005 | Subjects with Alzheimer's dementia, vascular dementia, or mixed dementia, in outpatient or residential settings, with NPI or NPI-NH score>5 on hallucination and delusion items<br>*Interventions:* placebo vs. flexibly dosed olanzapine (2.5–10 mg/day; mean dose: 5.2 mg/day) or risperidone (0.5–2 mg/day; mean dose: 1.0 mg/day)<br>*Design:* double-blind randomized trial<br>Industry-sponsored multicenter trial in the United States | 494 subjects, with 94 receiving placebo, 204 receiving olanzapine, and 196 receiving risperidone | 10 weeks | Risperidone vs. placebo: total SMD=−0.13 (−0.38, 0.12); psychosis SMD=−0.03 (−0.34, 0.16); agitation SMD= 0.14 (−0.11, 0.39) | 2 |

| Study type | Study | How subjects were recruited and what intervention(s) were performed[a] | Sample size[b] | How long subjects were followed | Outcome measures and main results | Rating of quality of evidence |
|---|---|---|---|---|---|---|
| 1A | De Deyn et al. 1999 | Hospitalized or institutional-ized individuals with MMSE score<24 and BEHAVE-AD score>7<br>*Interventions:* placebo vs. flexi-bly dosed haloperidol (0.5–4 mg/day; mean dose: 1.2 mg/day) or risperidone (0.5–4 mg/day; mean dose: 1.1 mg/day)<br>*Design:* randomized trial<br>Industry-sponsored multi-center trial in the United King-dom and Europe | 344 subjects; 68 of the 115 sub-jects receiving risperidone, 81 of the 115 sub-jects receiving haloperidol, and 74 of the 114 sub-jects receiving placebo com-pleted the trial | 12 weeks | Risperidone vs. placebo: total SMD=0.12 (−0.14, 0.38); agitation SMD= 0.31 (0.05, 0.57) | 4 |
| 1A | Katz et al. 1999 | Subjects with DSM-IV diagnosis of Alzheimer's disease, vascu-lar dementia, or mixed demen-tia, residing in a nursing home or chronic care facility, with MMSE score<24 and signifi-cant psychotic and behavioral symptoms (BEHAVE-AD score>7)<br>*Interventions:* placebo vs. fixed doses of risperidone (0.5, 1, or 2 mg/day)<br>*Design:* double-blind random-ized controlled trial<br>Industry-sponsored multi-center trial conducted in the United States | 625 subjects; 70% of the sub-jects completed the study | 12 weeks | Risperidone vs. placebo: total SMD=0.32 (0.11, 0.53); psychosis SMD=0.20 (−0.01, 0.41); agitation SMD= 0.38 (0.17, 0.60) | 4 |
| 1A | Mintzer et al. 2006 | Subjects with presentation that met criteria for Alzheimer's dementia (MMSE scores 5–23), residing in nursing homes or a long-term care setting, who were mobile and had psychosis<br>*Interventions:* placebo vs. flexi-bly dosed risperidone (0.5-1.5 mg/day; mean dose: 1.03 mg/day)<br>*Design:* randomized controlled trial<br>Industry-sponsored multi-center trial conducted in the United States | 473 subjects ran-domly assigned to treatment group, with 238 receiving placebo and 235 receiving risperidone; 354 subjects completed the study | 8 weeks, after 1–16 days of placebo run-in/washout | Risperidone vs. placebo: total SMD=−0.01 (−0.21, 0.18); psychosis SMD=0.17 (−0.02, 0.36); agitation SMD= 0.04 (−0.16, 0.23) | 3 |

| Study type | Study | How subjects were recruited and what intervention(s) were performed[a] | Sample size[b] | How long subjects were followed | Outcome measures and main results | Rating of quality of evidence |
|---|---|---|---|---|---|---|
| 1A | Schneider et al. 2006; Sultzer et al. 2008 | Subjects with Alzheimer's disease or probable Alzheimer's disease (MMSE scores 5–26), ambulatory and residing at home or in assisted living facilities, with moderate or greater levels of psychosis, aggression, or agitation *Interventions:* placebo vs. masked flexibly dosed olanzapine (mean dose: 5.5 mg/day), quetiapine (mean dose: 56.5 mg/day), or risperidone (mean dose: 1.0 mg/day) Stable doses of cholinesterase inhibitor were permitted. *Design:* multicenter, federally funded CATIE-AD trial—Phase 1 | 421 subjects randomly assigned to treatment group, with 142 receiving placebo, 100 receiving olanzapine, 94 receiving quetiapine, and 85 receiving risperidone | Median duration on Phase 1 treatment was 7.1 weeks; clinical outcomes assessed for those who continued to take antipsychotic at 12 weeks | Risperidone vs. placebo: total SMD=0.40 (0.13, 0.68); psychosis SMD=0.38 (0.11, 0.66); agitation SMD=0.10 (−0.17, 0.37) | 1 |

*Note.* 1=randomized controlled trial; 2=systematic review/meta-analysis; 3=observational; A=from AHRQ review. AHRQ=Agency for Healthcare Research and Quality; BEHAVE-AD=Behavioral Pathology in Alzheimer's Disease; CATIE-AD = Clinical Antipsychotic Trials of Intervention Effectiveness for Alzheimer's Disease; MMSE=Mini-Mental State Exam; NPI=Neuropsychiatric Inventory; NPI-NH=Neuropsychiatric Inventory—Nursing Home; SMD=standardized mean difference.
[a]Includes additional notes that may impact quality rating.
[b]Where applicable. Note overall *N* as well as group *n* for control and intervention.

### Quality of the Body of Research Evidence for Risperidone Versus Placebo in Psychotic Symptoms

*Risk of bias:* **Low**—Studies are all RCTs and vary in quality from low to high quality based on their described randomization and blinding procedures and their descriptions of study dropouts.

*Consistency:* **Inconsistent**—Effect sizes are overlapping, but four studies show an effect in the direction of risperidone benefit, with one study showing an effect in the direction of benefit for placebo. Two of the four studies showed a benefit of risperidone in psychosis that was statistically significant, but the other three studies did not show statistically significant benefit.

*Directness:* **Direct**—Studies measure overall BPSD, which is directly related to the PICOTS questions.

*Precision:* **Imprecise**—Confidence intervals vary in width, and the range of confidence intervals includes negative values in three studies.

*Applicability:* The included studies all involve individuals with dementia, including nursing home or hospital patients and non-institutionalized patients. Studies include subjects from around the world, including the United States, United Kingdom, Western Europe, and Australia/New Zealand. The doses of risperidone that were used in the studies are consistent with usual practice.

*Dose-response relationship:* **Absent**—One study examined different fixed doses of risperidone and appears to show a dose-response effect based on inspection of confidence intervals; however, these dose-response relationships did not show statistical differences across each pair of doses.

*Magnitude of effect:* **Weak effect**—The effect size is small but statistically significant.

*Confounding factors:* **Absent**—No known confounding factors are present that would be likely to reduce the effect of the intervention.

*Publication bias:* **Not suspected**—There is no specific evidence to suggest selection bias.

*Overall strength of evidence:* **Moderate**—The available studies of risperidone versus placebo are randomized trials of varying quality and have good sample sizes; however, the overall effect size of these trials is small according to the AHRQ meta-analysis. Four of the studies show benefit, and the benefit was statistically significant in two of the studies.

## Quality of the Body of Research Evidence for Second-Generation Antipsychotics Versus Placebo in Psychotic Symptoms

*Risk of bias:* **Low**—Studies are all RCTs, and the vast majority are double-blind trials. They vary in quality from low to high quality based on their described randomization and blinding procedures and their descriptions of study dropouts.

*Consistency:* **Inconsistent**—Effect sizes are generally overlapping, and the majority of the studies show an effect in the direction of SGA benefit. However, several studies showed no difference or favored placebo. On psychotic symptoms, the AHRQ meta-analysis shows small but statistically significant effects for risperidone only.

*Directness:* **Direct**—Studies measure psychosis, which is directly related to the PICOTS questions.

*Precision:* **Imprecise**—Confidence intervals for individual studies vary in size, and the range of confidence intervals includes negative values in the majority of studies.

*Applicability:* The included studies all involve individuals with dementia, including nursing home or hospital patients and non-institutionalized patients. The studies include subjects from around the world, including the United States, Canada, Western Europe, and Australia/New Zealand. The doses of SGA medications that were used in the studies are consistent with usual practice.

*Dose-response relationship:* **Absent**—For aripiprazole, quetiapine, and risperidone, only one study of each medication is available that assesses differing doses; two studies are available for olanzapine, with no consistency in results. There appear to be trends for dose-response relationships on measures of psychosis for aripiprazole and risperidone based on the confidence intervals, but these dose-response relationships did not show statistical differences across relevant pairs of doses.

*Magnitude of effect:* **Weak effect**—The effect sizes are small for all medications and significant only for risperidone.

*Confounding factors:* **Absent**—No known confounding factors are present that would be likely to reduce the effect of the intervention.

*Publication bias:* **Not suspected**—There is no specific evidence to suggest selection bias.

*Overall strength of evidence:* **Low**—A significant number of randomized trials of SGAs vs. placebo are available. Trials are of varying quality, but most have good sample sizes. However, there is a great deal of inconsistency in the study findings for individual medications and across the SGA medications as a whole.

## Overview and Quality of Individual Studies

TABLE A–23. **Overview of studies comparing olanzapine or quetiapine with risperidone for treating psychosis**

| Study type | Study | How subjects were recruited and what intervention(s) were performed[a] | Sample size[b] | How long subjects were followed | Outcome measures and main results | Rating of quality of evidence |
|---|---|---|---|---|---|---|
| 1A | Deberdt et al. 2005 | Subjects with Alzheimer's dementia, vascular dementia, or mixed dementia, in outpatient or residential settings, with NPI or NPI-NH score >5 on hallucination and delusion items. *Interventions:* placebo vs. flexibly dosed olanzapine (2.5–10 mg/day; mean dose: 5.2 mg/day) or risperidone (0.5–2 mg/day; mean dose: 1.0 mg/day). *Design:* double-blind, randomized trial. Industry-sponsored multicenter trial in the United States | 494 subjects, with 94 receiving placebo, 204 receiving olanzapine, and 196 receiving risperidone | 10 weeks | Olanzapine vs. risperidone: total SMD=0.10 (−0.10, 0.30); psychosis SMD=−0.03 (−0.23, 0.17); agitation SMD=−0.04 (−0.24, 0.16) | 2 |

**Overview of studies comparing olanzapine or quetiapine with risperidone for treating psychosis** *(continued)*

| Study type | Study | How subjects were recruited and what intervention(s) were performed[a] | Sample size[b] | How long subjects were followed | Outcome measures and main results | Rating of quality of evidence |
|---|---|---|---|---|---|---|
| 1A | Schneider et al. 2006; Sultzer et al. 2008 | Subjects with Alzheimer's disease or probable Alzheimer's disease (MMSE scores 5–26), ambulatory and residing at home or in assisted living facilities, with moderate or greater levels of psychosis, aggression, or agitation<br>*Interventions:* placebo vs. masked, flexibly dosed olanzapine (mean dose: 5.5 mg/day), quetiapine (mean dose: 56.5 mg/day), or risperidone (mean dose: 1.0 mg/day)<br>Stable doses of cholinesterase inhibitor were permitted.<br>*Design:* multicenter, federally funded CATIE-AD trial—Phase 1 | 421 subjects randomly assigned, with 142 receiving placebo, 100 receiving olanzapine, 94 receiving quetiapine, and 85 receiving risperidone | Median duration on Phase 1 treatment was 7.1 weeks; clinical outcomes assessed for those continuing to take antipsychotic at 12 weeks | Olanzapine vs. risperidone: total SMD=−0.27 (−0.56, 0.02); psychosis SMD= −0.27 (−0.56, 0.02); agitation SMD= −0.17 (−0.12, 0.16)<br>Quetiapine vs. risperidone: total SMD=−0.24 (−0.53, 0.06); psychosis SMD= −0.24 (−0.54, 0.05); agitation SMD= 0.10 (−0.20, 0.39) | 1 |

*Note.* 1=randomized controlled trial; 2=systematic review/meta-analysis; 3=observational; A=from AHRQ review.
AHRQ=Agency for Healthcare Research and Quality; CATIE-AD=Clinical Antipsychotic Trials of Intervention Effectiveness for Alzheimer's Disease; MMSE=Mini-Mental State Exam; NPI=Neuropsychiatric Inventory; NPI-NH=Neuropsychiatric Inventory—Nursing Home; SMD=standardized mean difference.
[a]Includes additional notes that may impact quality rating.
[b]Where applicable. Note overall *N* as well as group *n* for control and intervention.

## Quality of the Body of Research Evidence for Olanzapine or Quetiapine Versus Risperidone in Psychotic Symptoms

*Risk of bias:* **Low**—Studies are both RCTs but vary in quality from low to moderate based on their described randomization and blinding procedures and their descriptions of study dropouts.

*Consistency:* **Inconsistent**—Effect sizes are overlapping, but one study favors risperidone and the other study suggests no difference between risperidone and olanzapine.

*Directness:* **Direct**—Studies measure psychosis, which is directly related to the PICOTS questions.

*Precision:* **Imprecise**—Confidence intervals are wide, and the range of confidence intervals includes negative values in both studies.

*Applicability:* The included studies all involve individuals with dementia, including patients in institutional and outpatient settings. The studies include subjects from the United States. The doses of medication that were used in the studies are consistent with usual practice.

*Dose-response relationship:* **Not applicable to this comparison**.

*Magnitude of effect:* **Not applicable.**

*Confounding factors:* **Absent**—No known confounding factors are present that would be likely to reduce the effect of the intervention.

*Publication bias:* **Not suspected**—There is no specific evidence to suggest selection bias.

*Overall strength of evidence:* **Insufficient**—The available studies of risperidone as compared with olanzapine or quetiapine are randomized trials of low to moderate quality but have good sample sizes. However, the confidence intervals are relatively wide, and there is no consistency in the effect, and so it is difficult to draw conclusions with any degree of confidence.

## 2. Appropriate Dosage and Duration of Antipsychotic Treatment in Individuals With Alzheimer's Disease and Other Dementia Syndromes

Overview and Quality of Individual Studies

**TABLE A–24. Overview of studies on dose-related effects of second-generation antipsychotics in treating individuals with Alzheimer's disease and other dementia syndromes**

| Study type | Study | How subjects were recruited and what intervention(s) were performed[a] | Sample size[b] | How long subjects were followed | Outcome measures and main results | Rating of quality of evidence |
|---|---|---|---|---|---|---|
| 1A | Breder et al. 2004; Mintzer et al. 2007 | Nursing home residents with MMSE scores 6–22 and NPI or NPI-NH score >5 for hallucinations and delusions *Interventions:* placebo vs. three fixed doses of aripiprazole (2 mg, 5 mg, 10 mg) *Design:* double-blind randomized controlled trial Industry-sponsored multicenter trial conducted in long-term care facilities internationally, including the United States and Canada | 487 subjects enrolled; data for 284 analyzed | 10 weeks | Beginning at week 6 and continuing to study end point at week 10, subjects who received 10 mg aripiprazole daily had a statistically significant degree of improvement in NPI-NH Psychosis subscale scores as well as significant improvements in CMAI scores and scores on the NPI irritability, agitation/aggression, and anxiety items. A greater proportion of subjects who received aripiprazole 10 mg daily showed response to treatment (defined as a >50% decrease in NPI-NH Psychosis subscale scores from baseline) compared with subjects receiving placebo. Aripiprazole 5 mg/day differed from placebo in response rate and NPI subscores at early time points but not at 10 weeks, although CMAI scores remained improved. Response to aripiprazole 2 mg/day did not differ from response to placebo at any time point. | 1, 2 |

| Study type | Study | How subjects were recruited and what intervention(s) were performed[a] | Sample size[b] | How long subjects were followed | Outcome measures and main results | Rating of quality of evidence |
|---|---|---|---|---|---|---|
| 1A | De Deyn et al. 2004 | Subjects with Alzheimer's disease (MMSE scores 5–26), residing in long-term care settings, with hallucinations or delusions. *Interventions:* placebo vs. fixed-dose olanzapine (1, 2.5, 5, or 7.5 mg/day). *Design:* double-blind randomized trial. Industry-sponsored multicenter trial in Europe, Israel, Lebanon, Australia/New Zealand, and South Africa | 652 subjects; 65%–75% of the subjects in each study arm completed the trial | 10 weeks | No significant treatment effects, based on NPI-NH Psychosis Total and CGI-C scores, were seen at the 10-week end point for any of the doses of olanzapine. Repeated-measures analysis of the Psychosis Total scores showed significant within-group improvement from baseline in all five treatment groups. Nevertheless, a secondary comparison pooling across all visits showed a significant main effect of treatment with either 2.5 mg/day or 7.5 mg/day of olanzapine as compared with placebo. | 2 |
| 1A | Katz et al. 1999 | Subjects with DSM-IV diagnosis of Alzheimer's disease, vascular dementia, or mixed dementia, residing in nursing homes or chronic care facilities; with MMSE score <24 and significant psychotic and behavioral symptoms (BEHAVE-AD score >7). *Interventions:* placebo vs. fixed doses of risperidone (0.5, 1, or 2 mg/day). *Design:* double-blind randomized controlled trial. Industry-sponsored multicenter trial conducted in the United States | 625 subjects; 70% of the subjects completed the study | 12 weeks | Subjects who received either 1 mg/day or 2 mg/day of risperidone showed significant improvement relative to placebo on BEHAVE-AD Total scores and Psychosis and Aggressiveness subscale scores. These doses of risperidone remained superior to placebo on measures of aggressiveness after the study authors controlled for the effect of psychosis. | 4 |

| Study type | Study | How subjects were recruited and what intervention(s) were performed[a] | Sample size[b] | How long subjects were followed | Outcome measures and main results | Rating of quality of evidence |
|---|---|---|---|---|---|---|
| 1A | Street et al. 2000 | Subjects with possible or probable Alzheimer's disease, residing in nursing facilities, with NPI-NH score>2 *Interventions:* placebo vs. fixed doses of olanzapine (5, 10, or 15 mg/day) *Design:* double-blind randomized controlled trial Industry-sponsored multicenter trial conducted in the United States | 206 subjects; 66%–80% of individuals completed the trial in each study arm | 6 weeks | On the basis of the sum of the Agitation/Aggression, Hallucinations, and Delusions items of the NPI-NH, individuals receiving 5 mg/day or 10 mg/day of olanzapine had significant improvement relative to placebo, whereas those receiving 15 mg/day did not. A similar pattern of findings occurred in terms of the proportion of individuals who showed a response to treatment (as defined by at least a 50% reduction in score from baseline to end point) and in responses to the Psychosis and Agitation items. | 5 |
| 1A | Zhong et al. 2007 | Subjects with possible Alzheimer's disease or vascular dementia, in long-term care facilities, with agitation and PANSS-EC score>13 *Interventions:* placebo vs. quetiapine 100 mg vs. quetiapine 200 mg (dose adjusted according to fixed titration) *Design:* double-blind, randomized trial Industry-sponsored multicenter trial in the United States | 333 subjects | 10 weeks | There was a greater reduction from baseline to end point in mean PANSS-EC score with quetiapine 200 mg/day compared with placebo, but this difference in reduction was not significant using LOCF analysis. However, CGI-C scores were significantly improved with 200 mg/day quetiapine. At 100 mg/day, treatment with quetiapine did not differ from placebo. In terms of response (as defined by at least a 40% reduction on the PANSS-EC from baseline to end point), there were no differences among the treatment arms. | 2 |

*Note.* 1=randomized controlled trial; 2=systematic review/meta-analysis; 3=observational; A=from AHRQ review. AHRQ=Agency for Healthcare Research and Quality; BEHAVE-AD=Behavioral Pathology in Alzheimer's Disease; CGI-C=Clinical Global Impression of Change; CMAI=Cohen-Mansfield Anxiety Inventory; LOCF=last observation carried forward; MMSE=Mini-Mental State Exam; NPI=Neuropsychiatric Inventory; NPI-NH = Neuropsychiatric Inventory—Nursing Home; PANSS-EC=Positive and Negative Symptom Scale—Excitement Component; SMD=standardized mean difference.
[a]Includes additional notes that may impact quality rating.
[b]Where applicable. Note overall *N* as well as group *n* for control and intervention.

## Quality of the Body of Research Evidence for Dose-Related Effects of Second-Generation Antipsychotics

*Risk of bias:* **Low**—Studies are all RCTs and vary in quality from low to high quality based on their described randomization and blinding procedures and their descriptions of study dropouts.

*Consistency:* **Inconsistent**—Only a small number of studies include more than one dose of antipsychotic medication, and in the available studies, there is inconsistency regarding whether a dose response is present. Even in the studies for which confidence intervals suggest that a dose-response is present, these differences in dose generally do not reach statistical significance. There is overlap in the confidence intervals for the different doses in each study.

*Directness:* **Direct**—Studies measure overall BPSD, agitation/aggression, and psychosis, which are directly related to the PICOTS questions.

*Precision:* **Imprecise**—Confidence intervals vary in width, and the range of confidence intervals includes negative values in the majority of the studies.

*Applicability:* The included studies all involve individuals with dementia, with all of the studies involving nursing home patients. Although studies included subjects from around the world, including the United States, Canada, Western Europe, and Australia/New Zealand, the lack of inclusion of outpatients may limit its applicability.

*Dose-response relationship:* **Absent**—There appear to be trends for dose-response relationships on measures of global behavioral symptoms and psychosis for aripiprazole and risperidone and of agitation for risperidone, but these dose-response relationships did not show statistical differences across each pair of doses.

*Magnitude of effect:* **Not applicable**.

*Confounding factors:* **Absent**—No known confounding factors are present that would be likely to reduce the effect of the intervention.

*Publication bias:* **Not suspected**—There is no specific evidence to suggest selection bias.

*Overall strength of evidence:* **Insufficient**—Only one study is available that assesses differing doses for aripiprazole, quetiapine, and risperidone, and only two studies are available for olanzapine, with no consistency in results.

## 3. Effects of Specific Patient Characteristics on Effectiveness and Harms of Antipsychotic Medications in Individuals With Dementia

Available research evidence provides only limited data on the relative effectiveness and harms of SGAs for subsets of patients based on type of dementia, symptom severity, race/ethnicity, sex, or age. Although age, sex, and type of dementia are typically reported in describing the characteristics of study samples, these characteristics are rarely used in stratifying study results, although they are sometimes used in multivariate analyses of harms data in an effort to reduce experimental confounds. For example, one study (Rochon et al. 2013) found that men with dementia who were beginning treatment with an SGA were more likely than women to experience a serious adverse event, be hospitalized, or die within 30 days of treatment initiation (adjusted OR=1.47, 95% confidence interval [CI]=1.33–1.62). Another study (Marras et al. 2012), also using information from administrative databases found that men with dementia who were newly prescribed quetiapine, olanzapine, or risperidone were more likely to develop parkinsonism than women (adjusted HR=2.29,

95% CI=1.88, 2.79). On the other hand, women treated with antipsychotic medication were found to have more rapid cognitive declines than did men treated with antipsychotic medication in one study (Dutcher et al. 2014). Also, in the CATIE-AD trial (Zheng et al. 2009), significant weight gain was noted for women but not for men. In terms of symptom severity, individuals with a greater severity of BPSD may be at a higher risk of recurrent symptoms with discontinuation of antipsychotic medication (see "Discontinuation Studies" in section "1A. Efficacy and Comparative Effectiveness of Second-Generation Antipsychotics for Overall BPSD").

# 4. Potential Adverse Effects and/or Complications Involved With Prescribing Second-Generation Antipsychotics to Patients

The findings of the available evidence are summarized below for specific adverse effects. Although the strength of evidence ranges from high to insufficient for specific adverse effects, when the results are taken together, there is a high degree of confidence that several possible harms may be associated with antipsychotic use in individuals with dementia.

TABLE A–25. Strength of the available evidence for potential adverse effects with SGAs

| Adverse effect | Strength of evidence (from the 2011 AHRQ review[a]) | Summary of studies since the 2011 AHRQ review | Overall strength of evidence |
|---|---|---|---|
| Mortality | High for SGAs relative to placebo<br>Moderate for FGAs relative to SGAs | Moderate for FGAs relative to SGAs<br>Moderate for haloperidol relative to risperidone and for risperidone relative to quetiapine | High for SGAs relative to placebo<br>High for FGAs relative to SGAs<br>Moderate for haloperidol relative to risperidone and for risperidone relative to quetiapine |
| Stroke | Low | Low | Low |
| Myocardial infarction and other cardiovascular events | Low | Insufficient | Low |
| Pulmonary-related adverse effects | Insufficient | Low | Low |
| Cognitive changes | Low | Insufficient | Low |
| Sedation/fatigue | Moderate | N/A | Moderate |
| Extrapyramidal side effects (excluding tardive dyskinesia) | Moderate | Low | Moderate |
| Tardive dyskinesia | Insufficient | N/A | Insufficient |
| Falls and hip fractures | Insufficient | Low | Low |
| Development of diabetes | Low | Insufficient | Low |
| Weight gain | Moderate for elderly and those with dementia<br>High for all uses and ages | N/A | Moderate |
| Urinary symptoms | Low | N/A | Low |

Note.  FGA=first-generation antipsychotic; N/A=not applicable; SGA=second-generation antipsychotic.
[a]Maglione et al. 2011.

# Mortality

## Overview and Quality of Individual Studies

According to the 2011 AHRQ report, a well-conducted meta-analysis (Schneider et al. 2005), which was included in the 2006 AHRQ report, provided the best available estimate of risk of harm from mortality. This analysis, which included both published and unpublished trials, found that the use of SGAs (aripiprazole, olanzapine, quetiapine, or risperidone) is associated with an increased risk of death in patients with dementia and agitation, compared with placebo. The analysis showed a small but statistically significant difference in risk for death. For individual drugs, findings were not statistically significant; however, the absolute number of deaths with each drug was small, and the confidence intervals were wide, potentially obscuring an effect. Sensitivity analyses found no difference between the drugs.

TABLE A–26. **Pooled data on mortality from the 2011 AHRQ review**

| Adverse effect | Drug | Number of studies | Drug (adverse events/ sample size) | Placebo (adverse events/ sample size) | OR | (95% CI) | NNH |
|---|---|---|---|---|---|---|---|
| Death | Aripiprazole | 3 | 8/340 | 3/253 | 2.37 | (0.55, 14.18) | NC |
| Death | Olanzapine | 2 | 2/278 | 4/232 | 0.48 | (0.04, 3.62) | NC |
| Death | Quetiapine | 2 | 5/185 | 7/241 | 0.91 | (0.22, 3.41) | NC |
| Death | Risperidone | 5 | 39/1,561 | 17/916 | 1.19 | (0.63, 2.31) | NC |

*Note.* CI=confidence interval; NC=not calculated; NNH=number needed to harm; OR=odds ratio.
*Source.* Adapted from Maglione et al. 2011.

The authors of the 2011 AHRQ report (Maglione et al. 2011) reviewed six new, large high-quality cohort studies. These studies compared mortality in elderly patients taking second-generation and conventional antipsychotics. Taken together, the new studies suggested to the authors of the AHRQ report that conventional antipsychotics pose a same or higher degree of risk of death as SGAs. The authors characterized the strength of evidence for this outcome as moderate because the data were primarily from high-quality observational studies.

Since the AHRQ report, a large number of additional observational studies have been published that relate to the risk of mortality or serious adverse effects with antipsychotic treatment in the context of dementia. Data from these studies are consistent with the above conclusions of the AHRQ report in that the studies reported a greater risk of mortality with antipsychotics (first generation or second generation) and a same or higher degree of risk of death with first-generation as compared with second-generation agents. The majority of studies that examined mortality with FGAs reported data on haloperidol. Among the SGAs, data were most often reported for risperidone, olanzapine, quetiapine, and, less often, aripiprazole. Few studies reported on rates of mortality or serious adverse effects with ziprasidone. Relative to no antipsychotic treatment, a two- to threefold increase in mortality risk was typically seen with antipsychotic treatment, with statistically significant differences in most studies that showed higher mortality with FGAs as compared with SGAs. In comparisons of haloperidol and risperidone, there was typically an increase in risk of about 1.5-fold with haloperidol relative to risperidone. Comparisons among the other SGAs were less common, but a recent study (Maust et al. 2015) reported values for the number needed to harm (NNH) as 26 for haloperidol, 27 for risperidone, 40 for olanzapine, and 50 for quetiapine.

In the studies that address treatment duration and risk, the largest elevations in mortality were typically observed during the initial 120–180 days of treatment. Again, haloperidol and risperidone were most often studied, but similar patterns seemed to occur for olanzapine and quetiapine as well. Although a smaller number of studies assessed dose-effect relationship, higher doses of antipsychotic agents appeared to be associated with higher mortality risk.

In the observational studies there was typically a moderate risk of bias, and potential confounding factors were not always addressed. For example, the higher risk of death associated with the use of antipsychotics might have been because of patients' underlying neuropsychiatric symptoms (e.g., agitation) that prompted the use of antipsychotics rather than a direct effect of the agents. In studies that assessed this question, psychiatric factors such as the presence of psychosis or the severity of dementia were significantly associated with the time to death.

**TABLE A–27. Overview of studies examining risk of mortality with antipsychotics**

| Study type | Study | Subjects/Method/Design/Location | N | Duration | Outcomes/Results | Rating of quality of evidence |
|---|---|---|---|---|---|---|
| 3 | Chan et al. 2011 | Older adults with dementia residing in one of nine nursing homes *Design:* prospective cohort study *Location:* Hong Kong | 599 subjects | July 2009– December 2010; 18 months of follow-up | The 18-month rate for all-cause mortality in individuals exposed to an antipsychotic medication was 24.1%, while the rate in individuals not exposed to an antipsychotic was 27.5% ($P=0.38$). The exposed group also had a lower median rate of all-cause hospitalizations (56 [0–111] per 1,000 person-months vs. 111 [0–222] per 1,000 person-months), median (interquartile range), $P<0.001$. | 0 |
| 3 | Gardette et al. 2012 | Community-dwelling individuals with mild to moderate Alzheimer's dementia who were recruited from one of 16 memory centers *Design:* prospective cohort study *Location:* France | 534 total subjects; 102 of the subjects were new users of an antipsychotic agent during the follow-up period | 3.5-year follow-up period | 113 deaths occurred during the study. Use of either an FGA or an SGA was not an independent predictive factor of all-cause mortality after adjustment for dementia severity in multivariate analyses using a Cox proportional hazards model (HR=1.12; 95% CI: 0.59, 2.12). However, there was a suggestion of an increased risk of all-cause mortality with antipsychotic treatment in unadjusted and socio-demographically adjusted models. Common use of tiapride in this study may affect generalizability to U.S. patient populations. | 0 |

| Study type | Study | Subjects/Method/ Design/Location | N | Duration | Outcomes/Results | Rating of quality of evidence |
|---|---|---|---|---|---|---|
| 3 | Gerhard et al. 2014 | Subjects over 65 years of age who were living in the community and given a new prescription for risperidone, olanzapine, quetiapine, haloperidol, aripiprazole, or ziprasidone. Individuals with a prior diagnosis of schizophrenia, bipolar disorder, or cancer were not included. About one-third of individuals had a diagnosis of dementia, although the proportion of individuals with dementia was greater in those beginning treatment with risperidone, haloperidol, quetiapine, or ziprasidone than in those beginning treatment with olanzapine or aripiprazole. Data were obtained from U.S. Medicare or Medicaid claims databases. *Design:* retrospective cohort study *Location:* United States | 136,393 subjects, with 36.2% of the subjects receiving risperidone, 32.5% receiving olanzapine, 19.2% receiving quetiapine, 9.6% receiving haloperidol, 1.4% receiving aripiprazole, and 1.1% receiving ziprasidone | January 1, 2001– December 31, 2005 | Using Cox proportional hazards models to control for dose and propensity score, the study authors found that 180-day mortality risk was increased for haloperidol (HR=1.18; 95% CI: 1.06, 1.33) and decreased for quetiapine (HR=0.81; 95% CI: 0.73, 0.89) and olanzapine (HR=0.82; 95% CI: 0.74, 0.90) relative to risperidone. A similar pattern of findings was observed for specific causes of mortality (e.g., circulatory, cerebrovascular, respiratory). Overall noncancer mortality rate for the sample was 13.6 per 100 person-years (4,216 noncancer deaths, with an additional 180 cancer-related deaths). Unadjusted mortality rates ranged from 31.4 (95% CI: 29.1, 33.7) per 100 person-years for haloperidol to 5.8 (95% CI: 3.5, 8.1) per 100 person-years for aripiprazole. However, haloperidol was given at a higher average dose than were the other agents, and risperidone, olanzapine, and haloperidol each showed a dose–response relationship to mortality risk. (Sample sizes were insufficient to perform such calculation for other agents except quetiapine, which showed no dose-response relationship.) Inclusion of individuals who did not have a diagnosis of dementia limits generalizability. | 0 |

| Study type | Study | Subjects/Method/ Design/Location | N | Duration | Outcomes/Results | Rating of quality of evidence |
|---|---|---|---|---|---|---|
| 3A | Gill et al. 2007 | Subjects over 66 years of age with a diagnosis of dementia who were living in the community or in long-term care and who were identified through Ontario Health Insurance Plan or Discharge Abstract Databases as a new user of antipsychotic medication<br>*Design:* population-based, retrospective cohort study<br>*Location:* Canada | 27,259 pairs of individuals matched on the basis of propensity scores | April 1, 1997–March 31, 2002 | In both community-dwelling and long-term care–dwelling individuals, initiating use of an SGA was associated with a significant increase in the risk of death within 30 days as compared with nonuse (adjusted HR = 1.31 [95% CI: 1.02, 1.70] for community-dwelling individuals and 1.55 [95% CI: 1.15, 2.07] for individuals living in long-term care facilities) in multivariate analyses. Corresponding values for absolute risk difference were 0.2% and 1.2%, respectively. Mortality risk remained elevated at 180 days after treatment initiation. Use of an FGA medication was associated with a higher risk of mortality at 30 days than use of an SGA (adjusted HR=1.55 [95% CI: 1.19, 2.02] for community-dwelling individuals and 1.26 [95% CI: 1.04, 1.53] for individuals living in long-term care facilities). As with initiation of an SGA, this increase in risk was still present at 180 days after initiation of treatment. | 0 |

| Study type | Study | Subjects/Method/Design/Location | N | Duration | Outcomes/Results | Rating of quality of evidence |
|---|---|---|---|---|---|---|
| 3 | Gisev et al. 2012 | Individuals who were residing in a specific city in Finland on January 1, 2000 and were at least 65 years of age<br><br>Data were obtained from the Finnish National Prescription Register with information on diagnoses obtained from the Special Reimbursement Register.<br><br>*Design:* population-based retrospective cohort study<br>*Location:* Leppävirta, Finland | 2,224 subjects; 332 of the subjects used an antipsychotic medication during the study period. | Follow-up from 2000 to 2008 | Using time-dependent Cox proportional hazard models to assess all-cause mortality, the study authors found that the unadjusted HR for risk of death associated with antipsychotic use was 2.71 (95% CI: 2.3, 3.2). After adjustment for baseline age, sex, antidepressant use, and diagnostic confounders, the HR was 2.07 (95% CI: 1.73, 2.47). Adjusted HR was the highest among antipsychotic users with baseline respiratory disease (HR=2.21; 95% CI: 1.30, 3.76).<br><br>Inclusion of individuals who did not have a diagnosis of dementia may limit generalizability. | 0 |
| 3 | Hollis et al. 2007* | Subjects age 65 years or older who were taking or had initiated treatment with an antipsychotic, sodium valproate, or carbamazepine<br><br>Subjects identified through a database of prescriptions written for veterans or war widows.<br><br>*Design:* retrospective population-based cohort<br>*Location:* Australia<br>*Funding:* Australian Department of Veterans Affairs | 16,634 subjects initiated treatment during the study period, and 9,831 individuals continued treatment with one of the study medications. | 2003–2004 | Using mortality rates, Kaplan-Meier survival analysis, and adjusted Cox proportional hazards analysis, the study authors found that those initiating treatment with haloperidol, chlorpromazine, or risperidone had an increased relative risk of mortality compared with olanzapine (2.26 [95% CI: 2.08, 2.47]; 1.39 [95% CI: 1.15, 1.67], and 1.28 [95% CI: 1.07, 1.40], respectively). For those receiving continued treatment, relative risks of mortality compared with olanzapine were increased for haloperidol (1.38 [95% CI: 1.23, 1.54]) and risperidone (1.24 [95%: 1.10, 1.46]). | 0 |

| Study type | Study | Subjects/Method/ Design/Location | N | Duration | Outcomes/Results | Rating of quality of evidence |
|---|---|---|---|---|---|---|
| 3A | Huybrechts et al. 2011 | Nursing home residents age 65 years or older who had initiated treatment with psychotropics after admission *Study design:* retrospective population-based cohort *Location:* British Columbia | 10,900 subjects; 1,942 began treatment with an SGA, 1,902 began treatment with an FGA, 2,169 began treatment with an antidepressant, and 4,887 began treatment with a benzodiazepine. | 1996–2006 | Using proportional hazards models with propensity-score adjustments, the study authors found that users of FGAs had an increased risk of death (RR=1.47; 95% CI: 1.14, 1.91 for first generation), as compared with users of SGAs. Users of benzodiazepines also had a higher risk of death (RR=1.28; 95% CI: 1.04, 1.58) compared with users of SGAs. Using subgroup-adjusted propensity scores, individuals who began treatment with an FGA (as compared with users of an SGA) had an increased risk of mortality (RR=1.37; [95% CI: 0.96, 1.95] for individuals with dementia and 1.61 [95% CI: 1.10, 2.36] for individuals without dementia). Among individuals with no history of antipsychotic treatment, the corresponding RR was 1.33 (95% CI: 0.99, 1.77) as compared with users of an SGA. Inclusion of individuals who did not have a diagnosis of dementia may limit generalizability. | 0 |

| Study type | Study | Subjects/Method/ Design/Location | N | Duration | Outcomes/Results | Rating of quality of evidence |
|---|---|---|---|---|---|---|
| 3 | Huybrechts et al. 2012 | Nursing home residents with dementia age 65 years or older who were eligible for Medicaid and were new users of antipsychotic drugs (haloperidol, aripiprazole, olanzapine, quetiapine, risperidone, ziprasidone) Data were obtained from linked data from Medicaid, Medicare, MDS, National Death Index, and a national assessment of nursing home quality with propensity score adjustment used to control for potential confounders. *Design:* observational-retrospective cohort *Location:* United States | 75,445 subjects | 2001–2005 | Compared with users of risperidone, users of haloperidol had an increased 180-day risk of all-cause and cause-specific mortality (HR=2.07; 95% CI: 1.89, 2.26), and users of quetiapine had a decreased risk (HR=0.81; 95% CI: 0.75, 0.88). There was a dose-response relationship noted for all drugs except quetiapine, and the risk of mortality was increased with higher doses of medication. | 0 |
| 3A | Kales et al. 2007 | Subjects age 65 years or older who had a diagnosis of dementia and began outpatient treatment with an FGA or an SGA (risperidone, olanzapine, quetiapine, aripiprazole, ziprasidone, clozapine) Data were from Department of Veterans Affairs national database. *Design:* observational retrospective cohort *Location:* United States | 10,615 subjects | 2001–2005 | Mortality rates at 12 months did not differ for individuals treated with an SGA as compared with an FGA. Individuals treated with an antipsychotic had a higher rate of mortality at 12 months (22.6%–29.1%) as compared with those treated with non-antipsychotic medications (14.6%). | 0 |

| Study type | Study | Subjects/Method/ Design/Location | N | Duration | Outcomes/Results | Rating of quality of evidence |
|---|---|---|---|---|---|---|
| 3 | Kales et al. 2012 | Subjects age 65 years or older who had a diagnosis of dementia and began outpatient treatment with an antipsychotic (risperidone, olanzapine, quetiapine, or haloperidol) or valproic acid or its derivatives (as a non-antipsychotic comparison) Data were from Department of Veterans Affairs national database; data analyzed using multivariate models and propensity adjustments; covariate-adjusted intent-to-treat analyses; analyses were controlled for site of care and medication dosage *Design:* observational retrospective cohort *Location:* data obtained from the United States | 33,604 subjects | Fiscal years 1999–2008; compared 180-day mortality rates | In covariate-adjusted intent-to-treat analyses, haloperidol was associated with the highest mortality rates (relative risk=1.54; 95% CI: 1.38, 1.73) followed by risperidone (reference), olanzapine (relative risk=0.99; 95% CI: 0.89, 1.10), valproic acid and its derivatives (relative risk=0.91; 95% CI: 0.78, 1.06), and quetiapine (relative risk=0.73; 95% CI: 0.67, 0.80). Mortality risk with haloperidol was highest in the first 30 days but decreased significantly and sharply thereafter. Among the other agents, mortality risk differences were most significant in the first 120 days and declined in the subsequent 60 days during follow-up. | 0 |

| Study type | Study | Subjects/Method/Design/Location | N | Duration | Outcomes/Results | Rating of quality of evidence |
|---|---|---|---|---|---|---|
| 3 | Langballe et al. 2014 | Outpatients with dementia age 65 years or older who were prescribed antidementia drugs and psychotropic medications Subjects were identified through the Norwegian Prescription Database Study. *Design:* population-based cohort study *Location:* Norway | 26,940 subjects | 2004–2010 | Using Cox survival analyses, with adjustment for age, gender, mean daily defined dose, and severe medical conditions, the study authors found that antipsychotic use, as compared with use of other psychotropic agents, was associated with an approximately twofold increase in mortality at all studied time points after first dispensation (HR at 30 days=2.1 [95% CI: 1.6, 2.9] to HR at 730–2,400 days=1.7 [95% CI: 1.6, 1.9]). Haloperidol was associated with higher mortality risk (HR at 30 days=1.7 [95% CI: 1.0, 3.0] to HR at 730–2,400 days=1.4 [95% CI: 1.0, 1.9]) as compared with risperidone. | 0 |
| 3A | Liperoti et al. 2009 | Subjects with dementia over 65 years of age who were newly prescribed quetiapine, olanzapine, risperidone, clozapine, or an FGA Subjects were identified through the Systematic Assessment of Geriatric Drug Use via Epidemiology database (Medicare- or Medicaid-certified nursing facilities in five states in the United States). *Design:* observational-retrospective cohort *Location:* United States | 9,729 subjects | 1998–2000 | Rates of all-cause mortality were greater in individuals using FGAs as compared with those using SGAs (HR=1.26; 95% CI: 1.13, 1.42). | 0 |

| Study type | Study | Subjects/Method/ Design/Location | N | Duration | Outcomes/Results | Rating of quality of evidence |
|---|---|---|---|---|---|---|
| 3 | Lopez et al. 2013 | Outpatients with a diagnosis of probable Alzheimer's disease (of mild to moderate severity) who had at least one follow-up evaluation *Design:* observational cohort study *Location:* United States Funding: National Institute on Aging, National Institute of Mental Health | 957 subjects; 241 (25%) of the subjects were exposed to antipsychotics at some time during follow-up (138 to an FGA, 95 to an SGA, and 8 to both) | Mean follow-up time, 4.3 years (SD=2.7); range, 0.78–18.0 years | Death was more frequent in individuals taking an FGA than in individuals taking an SGA (69% vs. 34%, respectively). Nursing home admission was also more frequent in individuals taking an FGA than in individuals taking an SGA (63% vs. 23%, respectively). However, after adjusting for psychiatric symptoms using Cox proportional hazard models that adjusted for different combinations of age, gender, education level, dementia severity, hypertension, diabetes mellitus, heart disease, extrapyramidal signs, depression, psychosis, aggression, agitation, and dementia medication use, the study authors found that the associations between antipsychotic use and mortality or nursing home admission were no longer significant. Psychosis was strongly associated with nursing home admission and time to death. Neither FGAs nor SGAs were associated with time to death. | 0 |

| Study type | Study | Subjects/Method/ Design/Location | N | Duration | Outcomes/Results | Rating of quality of evidence |
|---|---|---|---|---|---|---|
| 3 | Maust et al. 2015 | Subjects age 65 years or older with a diagnosis of dementia Subjects were identified through a Veterans Health Administration database. *Design:* observational-retrospective case-control study *Location:* United States | 90,786 subjects; 46,008 of the subjects had received a new prescription for an antipsychotic (haloperidol, olanzapine, quetiapine, or risperidone), valproic acid and its derivatives, or an antidepressant | October 1, 1998– September 30, 2009 | In comparisons with respective matched nonusers of psychotropic medication, the increased mortality risk over 180 days of follow-up was 3.8% (95% CI: 1.0%, 6.6%; $P<0.01$), with an NNH of 26 (95% CI: 15, 99), in individuals receiving haloperidol; 3.7% (95% CI: 2.2%, 5.3%; $P<0.01$), with an NNH of 27 (95% CI: 19, 46), in individuals receiving risperidone; 2.5% (95% CI: 0.3%, 4.7%; $P=0.02$), with an NNH of 40 (95% CI: 21, 312), in individuals receiving olanzapine; and 2.0% (95% CI: 0.7%, 3.3%; $P<0.01$), with an NNH of 50 (95% CI: 30, 150), in individuals receiving quetiapine. In comparisons with antidepressant users, mortality risk ranged from 12.3% (95% CI: 8.6%, 16.0%; $P<0.01$), with an NNH of 8 (95% CI: 6, 12), for haloperidol users to 3.2% (95% CI: 1.6%, 4.9%; $P<0.01$), with an NNH of 31 (95% CI: 21, 62), for quetiapine users. As a group, SGAs (olanzapine, quetiapine, and risperidone) showed a dose-response increase in mortality risk, with 3.5% greater mortality (95% CI: 0.5%, 6.5%; $P=.02$) in the high-dose subgroup relative to the low-dose group. In direct comparisons with quetiapine, dose-adjusted mortality risk was increased with both risperidone (1.7%; 95% CI: 0.6%, 2.8%; $P=0.003$) and olanzapine (1.5%; 95% CI: 0.02%, 3.0%; $P=0.047$). | 0 |

| Study type | Study | Subjects/Method/ Design/Location | N | Duration | Outcomes/Results | Rating of quality of evidence |
|---|---|---|---|---|---|---|
| 3 | Musicco et al. 2011 | Subjects with dementia age 60 years or older who were newly prescribed an antidementia drug (donepezil, rivastigmine, or galantamine) Subjects were identified via the Italian Health Information System. *Design:* observational-retrospective cohort *Location:* Milan, Italy | All 4,369 residents of Milan (Italy) age 60 years or older who were newly prescribed an antidementia drug. All new users of antipsychotic drugs in this cohort were categorized according to whether antipsychotic was conventional ($n=156$) or second-generation ($n=806$), for a total of 962 subjects in this cohort taking antipsychotic drugs | January 2002– June 2008 | Mortality was increased two- and fivefold in users of SGAs and conventional antipsychotics, respectively, as compared with nonusers of antipsychotic medication. | 0 |
| 3 | Piersanti et al. 2014 | Outpatients with dementia over 65 years of age who were seen at an Alzheimer Evaluation Unit *Design:* observational-retrospective cohort *Location:* Italy | 696 individuals; 375 of the subjects were treated with an SGA (quetiapine, risperidone, or olanzapine) | January 2007– December 2009 | Relative risk of death in patients treated with SGAs was 2.354 (95% CI: 1.704, 3.279) as compared with subjects not treated with antipsychotic medication. Quetiapine was most commonly prescribed, and an association was seen between higher doses of this drug and higher mortality rates. | 0 |

| Study type | Study | Subjects/Method/ Design/Location | N | Duration | Outcomes/Results | Rating of quality of evidence |
|---|---|---|---|---|---|---|
| 3 | Rafaniello et al. 2014 | Subjects age 65 years or older who had dementia with behavioral and psychological symptoms and who were new users of SGAs and were seen at a Dementia Evaluation Unit *Design:* prospective cohort study *Location:* Italy | 1,618 subjects | Subjects enrolled between September 2006 and March 2010, with an average follow-up of 309 days | At least one adverse event was noted in 9.3% of the 1,618 new users of SGAs. Adverse effects included drug therapeutic failure (3.0%), extrapyramidal symptoms (0.5%), and stroke (0.2%). Death occurred in 5.1%, and the crude all-cause mortality rate was 6.0 per 100 person-years (95% CI: 4.8, 7.4). Mortality rates were higher in patients aged >85 years (9.0 per 100 person-years; 95% CI: 6.4, 12.7) and among male patients (7.5 per 100 person-years; 95% CI: 5.3, 10.6). In the multivariate analysis, only age was associated with all-cause mortality (HR=1.1 [95% CI: 1.0, 1.1] and 1.4 [95% CI: 0.9, 2.2], respectively), whereas hallucinations (HR=0.4; 95% CI: 0.2, 0.6) and dosage changes (HR=0.4; 95% CI: 0.2, 0.78) were associated with a significantly lower risk of all-cause mortality. | 0 |
| 3A | Rochon et al. 2008 | Subjects over 66 years of age with a diagnosis of dementia Subjects were identified via Ontario, Canada, administrative health care data. *Design:* observational-retrospective cohort *Location:* Ontario, Canada *Funding:* Canadian Institutes of Health Research | 20,682 community-dwelling and 20,559 nursing home–dwelling subjects | April 1, 1997 and March 31, 2004 | Likelihood of experiencing a serious adverse event (e.g., life-threatening, causing significant disability or death) was significantly greater in individuals treated with an FGA (3.8-fold increase; 95% CI: 3.31, 4.39) or SGA (3.2-fold increase; 95% CI: 2.77, 3.68) as compared with individuals who were not treated with an antipsychotic medication. | 0 |

| Study type | Study | Subjects/Method/Design/Location | N | Duration | Outcomes/Results | Rating of quality of evidence |
|---|---|---|---|---|---|---|
| 3 | Rochon et al. 2013 | Older adults with dementia who were newly prescribed oral SGA therapy; median age=84 years *Design:* observational-retrospective cohort *Location:* Ontario, Canada | 21,526 subjects (13,760 women, 7,766 men) | April 1, 2007, and March 1, 2010 | 1,889 subjects (8.8%) had a serious event, which was defined as a hospital admission or death within 30 days of treatment initiation (1,044 women, 7.6%; 845 men, 10.9%). Of these, 363 women (2.6%) and 355 men (4.6%) died. Men were more likely than women to be hospitalized or die during the 30-day follow-up period (adjusted OR=1.47, 95% CI: 1.33, 1.62) and consistently more likely to experience a serious event in each stratum. A gradient of risk according to drug dose was found for the development of a serious event in women and men. | 0 |
| 3A | Rossom et al. 2010 | Subjects over 65 years of age with a diagnosis of dementia Subjects were veterans identified through an administrative Veterans Health Administration National Patient Care Database. *Design:* observational-retrospective cohort *Location:* United States | 18,127 subjects (predominantly male) Subjects treated with antipsychotic (haloperidol [$n=2,217$], olanzapine [$n=3,384$], quetiapine [$n=4,277$], or risperidone [$n=8,249$]) were compared with those not taking an antipsychotic. | October 1999–September 2005 | During the initial 30 days of use, there was greater mortality in individuals exposed to haloperidol (5.4%), olanzapine (2.7%), or risperidone (2.8%), but not quetiapine (1.7%) as compared with individuals not taking an antipsychotic (1.7%), with unadjusted hazard ratios of 1.4, 1.6, 1.4, and 1.4, respectively. After the initial 30-day period, there was no difference in mortality among any of the antipsychotic-treated groups or when compared with individuals who did not receive treatment with an antipsychotic. | 0 |

| Study type | Study | Subjects/Method/ Design/Location | N | Duration | Outcomes/Results | Rating of quality of evidence |
|---|---|---|---|---|---|---|
| 3 | Rountree et al. 2012 | Subjects with probable Alzheimer's disease<br>*Design:* prospective cohort<br>*Location:* United States | 641 subjects | Mean follow-up time after the baseline visit to censoring or death: 3.0 (±1.94) years | Using multivariable Cox proportional hazard regression analysis, the study authors found that time-dependent changes in antipsychotic drug use, development of psychotic symptoms, antidementia drug use, and observed MMSE change were not predictive of time to death. Overall disease severity at baseline, medical comorbidities, and education also did not influence time to death. Baseline covariates significantly associated with increased survival were younger age ($P=0.0016$), female sex ($P=0.0001$), and a slower rate of initial cognitive decline from symptom onset to cohort entry ($P<0.0001$). Median survival time following the onset of symptoms was 11.3 years (95% CI: 10.4, 11.8). | 0 |

| Study type | Study | Subjects/Method/ Design/Location | N | Duration | Outcomes/Results | Rating of quality of evidence |
|---|---|---|---|---|---|---|
| 3A | Schnee-weiss et al. 2007; Setoguchi et al. 2008* | Subjects over 65 years of age who were being treated with an antipsychotic (risperidone, quetiapine, olanzapine, clozapine, or an FGA) Subjects were identified via a British Columbia Ministry of Health Pharmanet database. *Design:* observational-retrospective cohort *Location:* British Columbia, Canada *Funding:* government funded | 37,241 subjects were identified as meeting inclusion criteria; 12,882 of the identified subjects initiated treatment with an FGA, and 24,359 initiated treatment with an SGA. | January 1, 1996 to December 31, 2004 | Risk of death with FGAs was at least as high in terms of all-cause mortality as (and perhaps greater than) risk of death with SGAs (14.1% vs. 9.6%, mortality ratio 1.47 [95% CI: 1.39, 1.56]). Using multivariable and propensity score–adjusted modeling, the study authors found that the adjusted hazard ratio for mortality within 180 days of FGA initiation relative to SGA initiation was 1.27 (95% CI: 1.18, 1.37) for noncancer mortality, 1.23 (95% CI: 1.10, 1.36) for cardiovascular mortality, and 1.71 (95% CI: 1.35, 2.17) for respiratory mortality other than that due to pneumonia. Overall cardiovascular mortality and out-of-hospital cardiovascular mortality were each greater for doses of FGAs greater than the median prescribed dose. Hazard ratios for cardiovascular death with FGA as compared with SGA agents were also greatest in the initial days to weeks after treatment initiation. When data for individuals with dementia were analyzed separately, there was no difference in hazard ratios for overall cardiovascular mortality or for out-of-hospital cardiovascular mortality with FGAs as compared with SGAs (1.12 [95% CI: 0.80, 1.56] and 1.00 [95% CI: 1.22, 1.82], respectively). Inclusion of individuals who did not have a diagnosis of dementia may limit generalizability. | 0 |

| Study type | Study | Subjects/Method/ Design/Location | N | Duration | Outcomes/Results | Rating of quality of evidence |
|---|---|---|---|---|---|---|
| 3 | Simoni-Wastila et al. 2009 | Subjects who had stayed for at least 1 day in a long-term care facility Subjects identified based on data from a Medicare Current Beneficiary Survey. *Design:* retrospective cohort *Location:* United States *Funding:* government funded | 2,363 subjects; 742 of the subjects were treated with an antipsychotic during the first 6 months of a study year (194 were treated with an FGA and 456 with an SGA). | 1999–2002 | Using multiple Cox proportional hazards models and controlling for covariates, the study authors found that the adjusted hazard ratio for mortality with antipsychotic use relative to no antipsychotic use was 0.83 (95% CI: 0.69, 1.00) and was 0.89 (95% CI: 0.67, 1.19) for FGAs and 0.77 (95% CI: 0.62, 0.96) for SGAs analyzed separately. When the analysis was limited to individuals with a diagnosis of dementia, the adjusted hazard ratio was 0.77 (95% CI: 0.60, 0.98). | 0 |
| 3 | Sultana et al. 2014 | Subjects with vascular dementia Subjects were identified via anonymized versions of electronic health records from two National Health Service Foundation Trusts. *Design:* observational-retrospective cohort study *Location:* United Kingdom | 1,531 subjects; 337 of the subjects were exposed to quetiapine, risperidone, or olanzapine | 2007–2010 | No significant increases in mortality were noted in subjects exposed to SGAs (HR=1.05; 95% CI: 0.87, 1.26), risperidone (HR=0.85; 95% CI: 0.59, 1.24), or quetiapine (HR=1.14; 95% CI: 0.93, 1.39; $P$=0.20) compared with untreated patients. Too few patients were exposed to olanzapine alone to provide reliable results. | 0 |

**TABLE A–27. Overview of studies examining risk of mortality with antipsychotics (continued)**

| Study type | Study | Subjects/Method/Design/Location | N | Duration | Outcomes/Results | Rating of quality of evidence |
|---|---|---|---|---|---|---|
| 3 | Wang et al. 2005* | Subjects 65 years or older who initiated treatment with antipsychotic medication<br>Subjects identified through a drug insurance benefits database in Pennsylvania<br>*Design:* retrospective cohort study<br>*Location:* United States<br>*Funding:* government funded | 22,890 subjects; 9,142 initiated treatment with an FGA, and 13,748 initiated treatment with an SGA. | 1994–2003 | Within 180 days of antipsychotic initiation, mortality occurred in 17.9% of individuals treated with an FGA and in 14.6% of those treated with an SGA. Using Cox proportional hazards models, the study authors found that the adjusted hazard ratio for mortality with FGA as compared with SGA treatment was 1.37 (95% CI: 1.27, 1.49), with the highest hazard ratio in the initial 40 days of treatment (1.56 [95% CI: 1.37, 1.78]). For the subgroup of subjects with dementia, the adjusted hazard ratio for mortality with FGA as compared with SGA treatment was 1.29 (95% CI: 1.15, 1.45). | 0 |

*Note.* 1=randomized controlled trial; 2=systematic review/meta-analysis; 3=observational; A=from AHRQ review.
*Cited with other outcome.
AHRQ=Agency for Healthcare Research and Quality; CI=confidence interval; FGA=first-generation antipsychotic; HR=hazard ratio; MDS=Minimum Data Set; NNH=number needed to harm; NNT=number needed to treat; OR=odds ratio; RR=rate ratio; SGA=second-generation antipsychotic.

## Quality of the Body of Research Evidence for Harm Related to Mortality

*Risk of bias:* **Moderate**—Studies include 12 placebo-controlled RCTs with small numbers of deaths in each trial condition; mortality was not a primary outcome of these trials, which were designed to test efficacy. Mortality findings are also available from 26 observational studies, which are of low quality because of the lack of randomization, potential confounds of administrative database studies, and the lack of restriction of some studies to individuals with a presumptive diagnosis of dementia.

*Consistency:* **Consistent**—Pooled data from randomized, placebo-controlled trials did not show statistically significant differences in mortality when analyzed for each drug separately. However, the number of individuals in the pooled samples and the number of deaths in each of the treatment groups were relatively small. When placebo-controlled trial results were combined, SGAs had a small increase in mortality risk. In observational studies, 8 of 10 studies found an increase in the relative risk of mortality with antipsychotic use as compared with no antipsychotic use. In comparisons between FGAs and SGAs in terms of mortality, six studies showed an increase in mortality and one study showed a trend for increased mortality with FGAs that did not reach statistical significance. Four studies showed greater mortality with haloperidol than with risperidone and lower mortality with quetiapine than with risperidone. Other comparisons of mortality rates with specific antipsychotic medications showed mixed findings in observational studies.

*Directness:* **Direct**—Studies measure mortality, which is directly related to the PICOTS question on adverse effects.

*Precision:* **Imprecise**—Confidence intervals for the odds ratios from the pooled randomized data are relatively large, and the range of confidence intervals includes negative values. In the observational studies, there are also moderately wide confidence intervals on many of the reported hazard ratios, relative risks, and odds ratios.

*Applicability:* Many of the studies include individuals with dementia, although some of the administrative database studies included older individuals in nursing facilities without specifying a diagnosis. The doses of antipsychotic that were used in the randomized studies are consistent with usual practice. The randomized and observational studies include subjects from around the world, including the United States, United Kingdom, Canada, Finland, Italy, and Hong Kong. Randomized trials typically exclude individuals with significant co-occurring medical or psychiatric conditions as well as individuals who require urgent intervention before consent could be obtained, because inclusion of these individuals may influence the estimation of possible harms in broader groups of patients. For most of the observational studies, information about antipsychotic doses, co-occurring conditions, concomitant medications, and other factors that may influence applicability is unknown.

*Dose-response relationship:* **Present**—Two of the observational studies reported an effect of dose on mortality.

*Magnitude of effect:* **Weak effect**—The effect size is small in the majority of the observational studies. For the placebo-controlled studies, the results are not significant for individual medications but appear to vary by medication; the findings are significant when data were pooled in published meta-analyses.

*Confounding factors:* **Present**—The data from the observational studies have a number of potentially confounding factors. Because no information is available on co-occurring medical conditions in individuals receiving antipsychotic medications, these individuals may have been at greater risk of adverse outcomes independent of their use of antipsychotic medication. They also may have had a greater severity of dementia at the time of treatment, which could also impact adverse outcomes. There is also no way to determine whether the antipsychotic medications were given for delirium that was superimposed on dementia and delirium is known to be associated with increased risks of morbidity and mortality.

*Publication bias:* **Not suspected**—There is no specific evidence to suggest selection bias.

*Overall strength of evidence:* **High for SGA relative to placebo; high for FGA relative to SGA**; and **moderate for haloperidol relative to risperidone and for risperidone relative to quetiapine.**

## Cerebrovascular Accidents

### Overview and Quality of Individual Studies

The authors of the 2011 AHRQ report (Maglione et al. 2011) pooled data on cerebrovascular accidents (CVAs) from placebo-controlled trials and found that risperidone was the only drug associated with increased risk, as compared with placebo. As with data on mortality, the number of adverse events was small (20/1,479, or 1.4% for all placebo conditions, as compared with 35/1,902, or 1.8% for all the SGAs combined).

TABLE A–28. Pooled data on stroke and second-generation antipsychotic use from the AHRQ 2011 review

| Adverse effect | Drug | Number of studies | Drug (adverse events/ sample size) | Placebo (adverse events/ sample size) | OR | (95% CI) | NNH |
|---|---|---|---|---|---|---|---|
| Stroke | Aripiprazole | 3 | 2/340 | 2/253 | 0.70 | (0.05, 10.48) | NC |
| Stroke | Olanzapine | 2 | 6/278 | 4/232 | 1.46 | (0.33, 7.44) | NC |
| Stroke | Quetiapine | 2 | 3/185 | 6/241 | 0.65 | (0.10, 3.08) | NC |
| Stroke | Risperidone | 4 | 24/1,099 | 8/753 | 3.12 | (1.32, 8.21) | 53 |

*Note.* AHRQ=Agency for Healthcare Research and Quality; CI=confidence interval; NC=not calculated; NNH=number needed to harm; OR=odds ratio.
*Source.* Adapted from Maglione et al. 2011.

An industry-sponsored analysis of five randomized controlled trials of olanzapine in patients with dementia found that compared with patients taking placebo, patients taking olanzapine had a three times higher incidence of cerebrovascular adverse events. The AHRQ report authors found three studies that reported risk of stroke for antipsychotics. One of the studies reported that the risk was 12.4 times higher within the first month of antipsychotic use, as compared with nonuse. During subsequent months, the risk diminished and became insignificant. Another of the studies found that hospitalization was increased in the first week after use of a conventional antipsychotic. That study did not find the risk of stroke to be increased, however, by use of an SGA. The third study reported no difference in stroke risk between individuals treated with either an FGA or an SGA and those who received no treatment.

Since the 2011 AHRQ report, additional observational studies have examined the risks of cerebrovascular adverse events in patients with dementia who were being treated with antipsychotic agents. Of studies that compared risk in individuals receiving antipsychotic medication with those who did not receive an antipsychotic, five studies showed an increased risk of stroke (ranging from a 1.17-fold increase to a 12.4-fold increase in the initial month), whereas three studies showed no increase in the risk of stroke with antipsychotic treatment. Of the eight studies that compared an FGA with one or more SGAs, two studies showed an approximately 2-fold increase in risk of stroke with FGAs as compared with SGAs, whereas six studies showed no difference in risk, and one study showed greater risk with SGAs as compared with FGAs. As discussed in the section on mortality, these observational studies have a number of limitations, and the two studies that also assessed risk in individuals with or without dementia showed that the presence of dementia increased risk about 2-fold as compared with older individuals with no dementia.

**TABLE A–29.** Overview of studies examining risk of cerebrovascular accidents with antipsychotics *(continued)*

| Study type | Study | Subjects/Method/ Design/Location | N | Duration | Outcomes/Results | Rating of quality of evidence |
|---|---|---|---|---|---|---|
| 3 | Imfeld et al. 2013 | Subjects age 65 years or older with an incident diagnosis of Alzheimer's or vascular dementia, compared with a group of dementia-free patients. Subjects were identified from the United Kingdom–based General Practice Research Database. *Design:* nested case-control follow-up study *Location:* United Kingdom *Funding source:* unconditional pharmaceutical company grant | 18,729 subjects; 6,443 case subjects had Alzheimer's dementia, 2,302 had vascular dementia, and 9,984 had no dementia diagnosis | 1998 and 2008 | During the follow-up, there were 281 case subjects with incident ischemic stroke, 139 with hemorrhagic stroke, and 379 with a transient ischemic attack. The incidence rates of ischemic stroke for patients with Alzheimer's dementia, vascular dementia, or no dementia were 4.7/ 1,000 person-years (95% CI: 3.8, 5.9), 12.8/1,000 person-years (95% CI: 9.8, 16.8), and 5.1/1,000 person-years (95% CI: 4.3, 5.9), respectively. In comparison with dementia-free patients, the odds ratio of developing a transient ischemic attack when treated with SGAs was increased for patients with Alzheimer's dementia (OR=4.5; 95% CI: 2.1, 9.2) but not those with vascular dementia. | 0 |
| 3 | Kleijer et al. 2009 | Community-dwelling patients age 50 years or older who were prescribed at least one antipsychotic medication during the study period without having received an antipsychotic prescription for at least the preceding year Subjects were identified through Dutch community pharmacies and hospital discharge records. *Design:* nested case-control study *Location:* Netherlands *Funding:* no external funding | 26,157 individuals (mean age = 76 ± 9.7 years) met inclusion criteria; 518 of these individuals had a hospital admission for a cerebrovascular event and were matched by sex and age to four randomly selected individuals from the cohort | 1986–2003 | Current exposure and recent exposure to antipsychotics were associated with an increased risk of a cerebrovascular event compared with non-users (OR=1.7; 95% CI: 1.4, 2.2). A strong temporal relationship was found; the OR for a history of use less than a week is 9.9 (5.7–17.2). Risk decreases in time and is comparable to that for non-users after 3 months of use (OR=1.0; 95% CI: 0.7, 1.3). Inclusion of individuals who did not have a diagnosis of dementia limits generalizability. | 0 |

| Study type | Study | Subjects/Method/ Design/Location | N | Duration | Outcomes/Results | Rating of quality of evidence |
|---|---|---|---|---|---|---|
| 3 | Laredo et al. 2011 | Subjects age 65 years or older with a diagnosis of dementia who were prescribed an FGA or SGA Subjects were identified via electronic primary care records in the General Practice Research Database. *Design:* observational– case control *Location:* United Kingdom *Funding:* Foundation | 26,885 subjects; 3,149 of the subjects were eligible for the study and were matched to 15,613 control subjects | January 1, 1995– June 22, 2007 | After adjustment for confounding variables, the OR of a CVA associated with use of only FGAs versus no antipsychotic use in individuals with dementia age 65 or older was 1.16 (95% CI: 1.07, 1.27), and the OR for use of only SGAs versus no antipsychotics was 0.62 (95% CI: 0.53, 0.72). In the comparison of FGAs and SGAs, the OR was 1.83 (95% CI: 1.57, 2.14). FGAs appear to be associated with a higher risk of CVA, although the risk disappears with medication discontinuation. | 0 |
| 3 | Liperoti et al. 2005 | Subjects 65 years or older, residing in nursing facilities, with a diagnosis of dementia. Subjects were identified via Medicare data and the Systematic Assessment of Geriatric drug use via Epidemiology database. *Design:* retrospective, case-control *Location:* United States *Funding:* National Institutes of Health | 4,788 subjects; 1,130 of the subjects had been hospitalized for a stroke or transient ischemic attack; 3,658 control case subjects from the same facility had been hospitalized for septicemia or a urinary tract infection | June 30, 1998– December 27, 1999 | Using conditional logistic regression, the study authors found that users of antipsychotic medication did not have a significant difference in the odds ratio of being hospitalized for a cerebrovascular event as compared with non-users of antipsychotic medication. Odds ratio of a cerebrovascular event was 0.87 (95% CI: 0.67, 1.12) for risperidone, 1.32 (95% CI: 0.83, 2.11) for olanzapine, 1.57 (95% CI: 0.65, 3.82) for other SGAs, and 1.24 (95% CI: 0.95, 1.63) for FGAs. | 0 |

| Study type | Study | Subjects/Method/ Design/Location | N | Duration | Outcomes/Results | Rating of quality of evidence |
|---|---|---|---|---|---|---|
| 3 | Liu et al. 2013 | Subjects age 65 years or older who either had dementia with at least one inpatient service claim or at least two ambulatory care claims or were randomly chosen from the population as a sex-, age-, and index year–matched comparison subject<br>All subjects were identified using the Taiwanese Longitudinal Health Insurance Database for 2005.<br>*Design:* case-control<br>*Location:* Taiwan | 2,243 subjects with dementia; 1,450 of the subjects were treated with antipsychotic; 6,714 matched comparison subjects | 5 years of follow-up | Using Cox proportional-hazard regression, the study authors found that dementia patients had a twofold greater risk of developing stroke within 5 years of diagnosis compared with matched non-subjects, after adjustment for other risk factors (95% CI: 2.58, 3.08; $P<0.001$). Antipsychotic usage among patients with dementia increases risk of stroke 1.17-fold compared with patients without antipsychotic treatment (95% CI: 1.01, 1.40; $P<0.05$). | 0 |
| 3 | Percudani et al. 2005 | Subjects age 65 or older who had an inpatient admission for a cerebrovascular-related event<br>Subjects were identified via a national database of outpatient prescriptions with record linkage.<br>*Design:* retrospective population-based cohort<br>*Location:* Lombardy, Italy<br>*Funding:* not specified | 1,645,978 subjects; 36,075 of the subjects were exposed to an antipsychotic, with 9,265 exposed to an SGA | 2001 | Using logistic regression analysis, the study authors found that the odds ratio of a CVA in subjects receiving an antipsychotic was 1.24 (95% CI: 1.16, 1.32) relative to those not receiving an antipsychotic. Adjusted odds ratios were 1.42 (95% CI: 1.24, 1.69) for those receiving an SGA as compared with an FGA and 1.57 (95% CI: 1.08, 2.30) for those receiving risperidone as compared with haloperidol. No significant difference was noted in the odds ratio for CVA in those receiving clozapine, olanzapine, or quetiapine as compared with haloperidol.<br>Inclusion of individuals who did not have a diagnosis of dementia limits generalizability. | 0 |

| Study type | Study | Subjects/Method/Design/Location | N | Duration | Outcomes/Results | Rating of quality of evidence |
|---|---|---|---|---|---|---|
| 3A | Pratt et al. 2010 | Subjects over 65 years of age who were identified via an Australian Government Department of Veterans' Affairs database *Design:* observational, self-controlled case series *Location:* Australia | 10,638 subjects, with 514 receiving treatment that included initiation of an FGA and 564 receiving treatment that included initiation of an SGA | January 1, 2003– December 31, 2006 | In the first week after initiation of an FGA, there was an increased risk of hospital admission for stroke (IRR=2.3; 95% CI: 1.3, 3.8), whereas no such risk was seen after initiation of an SGA. Inclusion of individuals who did not have a diagnosis of dementia limits generalizability. | 0 |
| 3 | Sacchetti et al. 2008 | Subjects over 65 years of age identified via data from a health search database of primary care patients in Italy *Design:* observational-retrospective cohort *Location:* Italy *Funding:* Health Authority of the Lombardia Region | 69,939 identified as non-users of antipsychotic medication; 4,223 had received an initial antipsychotic prescription during the study period (599 with atypicals, 749 with butyrophenones, 907 with phenothiazines, and 1,968 with substituted benzamides) | January 2000– June 2003 | Crude incidence of stroke was 12.0/1,000 person-years for subjects not exposed to antipsychotic as compared with 47.1, 72.7, 25.0, and 47.4 per 1,000 person-years for those prescribed butyrophenones, phenothiazines, substituted benzamides, and SGAs, respectively. Using multivariate Cox proportional regression analysis, the study authors found that the adjusted risk ratio for stroke as compared with subjects without antipsychotic exposure was 5.79 (95% CI: 3.07, 10.9), 3.55 (95% CI: 1.56, 8.07), and 2.46 (95% CI: 1.07, 5.65) for butyrophenones, phenothiazines, and SGAs, respectively. As compared with SGAs, the adjusted risk ratio for stroke was 1.44 (95% CI: 0.55, 3.76) for butyrophenones and 2.34 (95% CI: 1.01, 5.41) for phenothiazines. Inclusion of individuals who did not have a diagnosis of dementia limits generalizability. | 0 |

| Study type | Study | Subjects/Method/ Design/Location | N | Duration | Outcomes/Results | Rating of quality of evidence |
|---|---|---|---|---|---|---|
| 3A | Sacchetti et al. 2010 | Subjects identified as being over 50 years of age based on data from a Health Search database of primary care patients in Italy *Design:* observational-retrospective cohort *Location:* Italy | 128,308 subjects (total who were identified as meeting inclusion criteria) | Not stated | Risk of stroke at the end of the first month of treatment was 12.4 times higher in individuals treated with antipsychotic as compared with those without antipsychotic exposure. However, absolute differences were small in terms of the cumulative proportion surviving (0.9921 [95% CI: 0.9899, 0.9943] with antipsychotic vs. 0.9995 [95% CI: 0.9979, 0.9983] without antipsychotic at 1 month; 0.9819 [95% CI: 0.9761, 0.9879] with antipsychotic vs. 0.9964 [95% CI: 0.9960, 0.9968] without antipsychotic at 6 months). | 0 |

*Note.* 1=randomized controlled trial; 2=systematic review/meta-analysis; 3=observational; A=from AHRQ review. AHRQ=Agency for Healthcare Research and Quality; CI=confidence interval; CVA=cardiovascular accident; FGA=first-generation antipsychotic; HR=hazard ratio; IRR=incidence rate ratio; OR=odds ratio; SGA=second-generation antipsychotic.

## Quality of the Body of Research Evidence for Harm Related to Cerebrovascular Accidents

*Risk of bias:* **Moderate**—Studies include 11 placebo-controlled RCTs with small numbers of CVAs in each trial condition. Harms of treatment were not a primary outcome of these trials, which were designed to test efficacy. Findings on the occurrence of CVAs are also available from 15 observational studies, which are of low quality due to the lack of randomization, potential confounds of administrative database studies, and the lack of restriction of some studies to individuals with a presumptive diagnosis of dementia.

*Consistency:* **Inconsistent**—With the exception of risperidone, pooled data from randomized placebo-controlled trials did not show statistically significant differences in CVA occurrence when analyzed for each drug separately. However, the number of individuals in the pooled samples and the number of CVAs in each of the treatment groups were relatively small. A separate industry-sponsored analysis, using pooled data, also showed an increase risk of CVA for olanzapine. When placebo-controlled trial results were combined, SGAs had a small increase in CVA risk. Of studies that compared risk in individuals receiving antipsychotic medication with risk in those who did not receive an antipsychotic, four of seven studies showed an increased risk of stroke. Of the nine studies that compared an FGA with one or more SGAs, two studies showed increased risk of stroke with FGAs as compared with SGAs, and one showed increased risk with SGAs as compared with FGAs.

*Directness:* **Direct**—Studies measure rates of CVAs, which are directly related to the PICOTS question on adverse effects.

*Precision:* **Imprecise**—Confidence intervals for the odds ratios from the pooled randomized data are relatively large, and the range of confidence intervals includes negative values in many cases. In the observational studies, there are also moderately wide confidence intervals on many of the reported hazard ratios, relative risks, and odds ratios.

*Applicability:* The included studies primarily involve individuals with dementia, although some of the administrative database studies included older individuals without specifying a diagnosis. The doses of antipsychotic that were used in the randomized studies are consistent with usual practice. The randomized and observational studies include subjects from around the world, including the United States, United Kingdom, Canada, Australia, Italy, Taiwan, and Hong Kong. It is not clear how many of the administrative database studies included nursing facility patients, and so its applicability may be limited. Randomized trials typically exclude individuals with significant co-occurring medical or psychiatric conditions as well as individuals who require urgent intervention before consent could be obtained, and this may influence the estimation of possible harms in broader groups of patients. For most of the observational studies, information about antipsychotic doses, co-occurring conditions, concomitant medications, and other factors that may influence applicability is unknown.

*Dose-response relationship:* **Unknown**—This was not assessed in the reported studies.

*Magnitude of effect:* **Weak effect**—The effect size is small in the majority of the observational studies. For the placebo-controlled studies, results are not significant for individual medications but appear to vary by medication; findings are significant when data were pooled in published meta-analyses.

*Confounding factors:* **Present**—The data from the observational studies have a number of potentially confounding factors. Because no information is available on co-occurring medical conditions in individuals receiving antipsychotic medications, these individuals may have been at greater risk of adverse outcomes independent of their use of antipsychotic medication. They also may have had a greater severity of dementia at the time of treatment, which could also impact adverse outcomes. Vascular disease has been reported to affect risk of CVA in some studies, and this is also not reported or accounted for in the RCTs or observational studies.

*Publication bias:* **Not suspected**—There is no specific evidence to suggest selection bias.

*Overall strength of evidence:* **Low.**

## Cardiovascular Events

### Overview and Quality of Individual Studies

From a meta-analysis using data from placebo-controlled trials on symptoms categorized as cardiovascular (including "cardiovascular symptoms," "edema," and "vasodilatation"), the authors of the 2011 AHRQ report (Maglione et al. 2011) noted that cardiovascular events were significantly more likely to occur among patients taking olanzapine or risperidone than among those taking placebo. However, no statistical association was shown between cardiovascular symptoms and treatment with either quetiapine or aripiprazole. Taken together, the rates of cardiovascular events were 230/3,256 (7.1%) for subjects who had received risperidone, olanzapine, quetiapine, or aripiprazole and 70/1,825 (3.8%) for subjects who had received placebo. An additional observational study also suggested an increased risk of myocardial infarction in the first 30–60 days of treatment. In terms of the relative risk of FGAs as compared with SGAs, one observational study showed no difference in risk of cardiovascular mortality in subjects who had a diagnosis of dementia.

## TABLE A–30. Pooled data on cardiovascular effects from the 2011 AHRQ review

| Adverse effect | Drug | Number of studies | Drug (adverse events/ sample size) | Placebo (adverse events/ sample size) | OR | (95% CI) | NNH |
|---|---|---|---|---|---|---|---|
| Cardiovascular | Aripiprazole | 1 | 42/366 | 12/121 | 1.18 | (0.58, 2.55) | NC |
| Cardiovascular | Olanzapine | 5 | 40/778 | 9/440 | 2.33 | (1.08, 5.61) | 48 |
| Cardiovascular | Quetiapine | 3 | 29/355 | 15/254 | 1.08 | (0.53, 2.30) | NC |
| Cardiovascular | Risperidone | 6 | 119/1,757 | 34/1,010 | 2.08 | (1.38, 3.22) | 34 |

*Note.* AHRQ=Agency for Healthcare Research and Quality; CI=confidence interval; NC=not calculated; NNH=number needed to harm; OR=odds ratio.
*Source.* Adapted from Maglione et al. 2011.

## TABLE A–31. Overview of studies examining risk of cardiovascular events with antipsychotics

| Study type | Study | Subject/Method/ Design/Location | N | Duration | Outcomes/Results | Rating of quality of evidence |
|---|---|---|---|---|---|---|
| 3 | Pariente et al. 2012 | Older community-dwelling patients who began treatment with a cholinesterase inhibitor treatment Subjects were identified via the Quebec, Canada, prescription claims database. *Design:* observational-retrospective cohort *Location:* Quebec, Canada | 37,138 subjects; 10,969 (29.5%) of the subjects started antipsychotic treatment during the follow-up period and were matched with a sample of individuals who did not use antipsychotic medications. | January 1, 2000– December 31, 2009 | Of individuals who started taking antipsychotic medication, 1.3% of them had an MI within the initial year of treatment. Hazard ratios were 2.19 (95% CI: 1.11, 4.32) for the first 30 days, 1.62 (95% CI: 0.99, 2.65) for the first 60 days, 1.36 (95% CI: 0.89, 2.08) for the first 90 days, and 1.15 (95% CI: 0.89, 1.47) for the first 365 days based on Cox proportional hazards models, with adjustment for age, sex, cardiovascular risk factors, psychotropic drug use, and propensity scores. A self-controlled case series study using Poisson regression in 804 instances of MI in new users of antipsychotic showed IRRs of 1.78 (95% CI: 1.26, 2.52) for 1–30 days, 1.67 (95% CI: 1.09, 2.56) for 31–60 days, and 1.37 (95% CI: 0.82, 2.28) for 61–90 days. | 0 |

TABLE A–31. **Overview of studies examining risk of cardiovascular events with antipsychotics** *(continued)*

| Study type | Study | Subject/Method/Design/Location | N | Duration | Outcomes/Results | Rating of quality of evidence |
|---|---|---|---|---|---|---|
| 3A | Schnee-weiss et al. 2007; Setogu-chi et al. 2008* | Subjects over 65 years of age who were being treated with an antipsy-chotic (risperidone, quetiapine, olan-zapine, clozapine, or FGA) Subjects were identi-fied via data from a British Columbia Ministry of Health Pharmanet data-base. *Design:* observa-tional-retrospec-tive cohort *Location:* British Columbia, Canada *Funding:* govern-ment funded | 37,241 subjects identified as meeting inclu-sion criteria; 12,882 of the identified sub-jects initiated treatment with an FGA, and 24,359 initiated treatment with an SGA | January 1, 1996 to December 31, 2004 | Using multivariable and propen-sity score–adjusted modeling, the study authors found that the adjusted hazard ratio for mortal-ity within 180 days of FGA initi-ation relative to SGA initiation was 1.23 (95% CI: 1.10, 1.36) for cardiovascular mortality. Over-all cardiovascular mortality and out-of-hospital cardiovascular mortality were each greater for doses of FGAs greater than the median prescribed dose. Hazard ratios for cardiovascular death with FGAs as compared with SGAs were also greatest in the initial days to weeks after treat-ment initiation. When data for individuals with dementia were analyzed separately, there was no difference in hazard ratios for overall cardiovascular mortality or for out-of-hospital cardiovas-cular mortality with FGAs as compared with SGAs (1.12 [95% CI: 0.80, 1.56] and 1.00 [95% CI: 1.22, 1.82], respectively). Inclusion of some individuals who did not have a diagnosis of dementia may limit generaliz-ability. | 0 |

*Note.* 1=randomized controlled trial; 2=systematic review/meta-analysis; 3=observational; A=from AHRQ review.
*Cited with other outcome.
AHRQ=Agency for Healthcare Research and Quality; CI=confidence interval; FGA=first-generation antipsychotic; IRR=incidence rate ratio; MI=myocardial infarction; SGA=second-generation antipsychotic.

## Quality of the Body of Research Evidence for Harm Related to Cardiovascular Events

*Risk of bias:* **Moderate**—Studies include placebo-controlled RCTs, but cardiovascular events were not a primary outcome of these trials, which were designed to test efficacy. Also, the category of cardiovascular events includes multiple different adverse effects, which are likely to have different degrees of risk and different mechanisms. Findings from the two observational studies are of low quality due to the lack of randomization.

*Consistency:* **Consistent**—Across the SGAs as a group, there was a consistent increase in risk of a cardiovascular event with antipsychotic treatment. Among the SGAs, increased rates of cardiovas-cular events were noted for olanzapine and risperidone, but not quetiapine or olanzapine, in the pooled findings from RCTs. One observational study showed an increased risk of cardiovascular events in new users of antipsychotic medication. Another observational study also showed an increased risk in elderly users of FGAs as compared with SGAs, although no increase in risk was noted when data analysis was restricted to individuals with dementia.

*Directness:* **Direct**—Studies measure rates of cardiovascular events, which are directly related to the PICOTS question on adverse effects.

*Precision:* **Precise**—Confidence intervals for the odds ratios from the pooled randomized data are moderate in size, as are the incidence rate ratios from the available observational study.

*Applicability:* The included studies involve individuals with dementia. The doses of antipsychotic that were used in the randomized studies are consistent with usual practice. The randomized studies include subjects from many countries, whereas the administrative data from the observational studies are from Canada. It is not clear how many of the RCT studies included nursing facility patients, and so applicability may be limited because the observational study was only conducted in a community sample. Randomized trials typically exclude individuals with significant co-occurring medical or psychiatric conditions as well as individuals who require urgent intervention before consent could be obtained, and this may influence the estimation of possible harms in broader groups of patients. For the observational studies, information about antipsychotic doses, co-occurring conditions, concomitant medications, and other factors that may influence applicability is unclear.

*Dose-response relationship:* **Unknown**—This was not assessed in the reported studies.

*Magnitude of effect:* **Weak effect**—The effect size is small based on the pooled odds ratios in the placebo-controlled studies; however, results appear to vary by medication.

*Confounding factors:* **Present**—The data from the observational studies have a number of potentially confounding factors. Because no information is available on co-occurring medical conditions in individuals receiving antipsychotic medications, these individuals may have been at greater risk of adverse outcomes independent of their use of antipsychotic medication. They also may have had a greater severity of dementia at the time of treatment, which could also impact adverse outcomes. The decreasing degree of risk with time that was seen in the observational study may be due to an intercurrent process that prompts antipsychotic use rather than an outgrowth of antipsychotic treatment.

*Publication bias:* **Not suspected**—There is no specific evidence to suggest selection bias.

*Overall strength of evidence:* **Low**.

## Pulmonary-Related Adverse Events

### Overview and Quality of Individual Studies

The authors of the AHRQ report (Maglione et al. 2011) noted small numbers of pulmonary events in single RCTs of quetiapine and ziprasidone, with no statistically significant differences between placebo and treatment with that limited evidence base.

| Adverse effect | Drug | Number of studies | Drug (adverse events/ sample size) | Placebo (adverse events/ sample size) | OR | (95% CI) | NNH |
|---|---|---|---|---|---|---|---|
| Pulmonary | Aripiprazole | 1 | 6/106 | 3/102 | 1.97 | (0.41, 12.54) | NC |
| Pulmonary | Olanzapine | 1 | 0/204 | 3/94 | 0.00 | (0.00, 1.10) | NC |
| Pulmonary | Risperidone | 1 | 6/196 | 3/94 | 0.96 | (0.20, 6.05) | NC |

*Note.* AHRQ=Agency for Healthcare Research and Quality; CI=confidence interval; NC=not calculated; NNH=number needed to harm; OR=odds ratio.
*Source.* Adapted from Maglione et al. 2011.

In one head-to-head trial, one patient treated with risperidone had a pulmonary adverse event, compared with no one in the olanzapine group. In observational studies, three studies reported increases in the risk of pneumonia for individuals with dementia treated with antipsychotic agents. In one study the risk was only seen for SGAs but appeared to be dose-dependent. In the other two studies the risk was comparable for FGAs as compared with SGAs, but in one of these studies the period of increased risk began before the antipsychotic medication was initiated. In an additional study of individuals 65 years and older, there was an increase in the likelihood of pneumonia in individuals receiving an antipsychotic, but no information was available on whether subjects had a diagnosis of dementia.

Overall, risk was highest early in the studies and declined with time. One observational study showed an increased risk of nonpneumonia respiratory mortality with FGAs as compared with SGAs among individuals over age 65. One observational study showed an approximately 1.5-fold increase in the risk of venous thromboembolism (VTE) with new use of an antipsychotic.

TABLE A–33. Overview of studies examining risk of pulmonary-related adverse events with antipsychotics

| Study type | Study | Subject/Method/ Design/Location | N | Duration | Outcomes/Results | Rating of quality of evidence |
|---|---|---|---|---|---|---|
| 3A | Huybrechts et al. 2011* | Nursing home residents age 65 years or older who had treatment with psychotropics initiated after admission. *Design:* retrospective population-based cohort. *Location:* British Columbia | 10,900 individuals; 1,942 of the subjects started taking an SGA, 1,902 started taking an FGA, 2,169 started taking an antidepressant, and 4,887 started taking a benzodiazepine | 1996–2006 | There was no difference observed in the risk of heart failure or pneumonia in individuals receiving FGAs, as compared with SGAs, with RR of 1.03 (95% CI: 0.62, 1.69) and 0.91 (95% CI: 0.41, 2.01), respectively. Inclusion of individuals who did not have a diagnosis of dementia may limit generalizability. | 0 |

**Overview of studies examining risk of pulmonary-related adverse events with antipsychotics** *(continued)*

| Study type | Study | Subject/Method/Design/Location | N | Duration | Outcomes/Results | Rating of quality of evidence |
|---|---|---|---|---|---|---|
| 3 | Knol et al. 2008 | Community-dwelling subjects, age 65 or older, who had been exposed to antipsychotic medication Subjects identified via a national pharmacy database. *Design:* observational-retrospective nested case control study *Location:* Netherlands *Funding:* no industry funding | 22,944 subjects received an antipsychotic during the study period; 543 of these subjects had a hospitalization for pneumonia, and 2,163 randomly selected individuals served as controls | April 1985– December 2003 | Using multivariate logistic regression, the study authors found that current use of an antipsychotic as compared with no prior antipsychotic use was associated with an increased likelihood of hospitalization for pneumonia (adjusted odds ratio=1.6; 95% CI: 1.3, 2.1), whereas past use of an antipsychotic did not show an effect. Lack of information about dementia diagnosis may limit generalizability. | 0 |
| 3* | Pratt et al. 2011 | Subjects over 65 years of age who were exposed to antipsychotic medication Subjects identified via the Australian Department of Veterans' Affairs Health Care Claims Database. *Design:* observational-retrospective cohort *Location:* Australia *Funding:* Australian Government | 8,235 subjects had at least one hospitalization for hip fracture, and of these 494 had begun receiving an FGA and 1,091 had begun receiving an SGA; 13,324 had at least one hospitalization for pneumonia, and of these 807 had begun receiving an FGA and 1,107 had begun receiving an SGA during the study period | 2005–2008; median follow-up: 3.3–4.0 years | Using a self-controlled case-series design, the study authors found that the risk of hospitalization for pneumonia was increased during all post-exposure periods for both FGA and SGA and remained significantly increased with more than 12 weeks of continuous exposure (IRR=1.43; 95% CI: 1.23, 1.66). Risk of pneumonia was elevated for up to 12 weeks prior to the initiation of FGAs or SGAs. | 0 |

| Study type | Study | Subject/Method/ Design/Location | N | Duration | Outcomes/Results | Rating of quality of evidence |
|---|---|---|---|---|---|---|
| 3 | Schmedt and Garbe 2013 | Subjects age 65 years or older with dementia Subjects were identified via the German Pharmacoepidemiological Research Database. *Design:* nested case-control study *Location:* Germany *Funding:* no pharmaceutical funding | 72,591 individuals in total cohort, from which there were 1,028 VTE cases and 4,109 controls matched to each case according to age, sex, health insurance, and calendar time of the VTE | 2004–2007 | Using multivariate conditional logistic regression, the study authors found an increased risk of VTE for current users of antipsychotic medication (OR=1.23; 95% CI: 1.01–1.50) and for users of a combination of an FGA and an SGA (OR=1.62; 95% CI: 1.15, 2.27). In current users, only new use was associated with an increased risk (OR=1.63; 95% CI: 1.10, 2.40). | 0 |
| 3A | Schneeweiss et al. 2007; Setoguchi et al. 2008* | Subjects over 65 years of age who were being treated with an antipsychotic (risperidone, quetiapine, olanzapine, clozapine, or FGA) Subjects were identified via data from a British Columbia Ministry of Health Pharmanet database. *Design:* observational-retrospective cohort *Location:* British Columbia, Canada *Funding:* government funded | 37,241 subjects identified as meeting inclusion criteria; 12,882 of the identified subjects initiated treatment with an FGA, and 24,359 initiated treatment with an SGA | January 1, 1996 to December 31, 2004 | Using multivariable and propensity score–adjusted modeling, the study authors found that the adjusted hazard ratio for mortality within 180 days of FGA initiation relative to SGA initiation was 1.71 (95% CI: 1.35, 2.17) for respiratory mortality other than that due to pneumonia. Inclusion of individuals who did not have a diagnosis of dementia may limit generalizability. | 0 |

| Study type | Study | Subject/Method/ Design/Location | N | Duration | Outcomes/Results | Rating of quality of evidence |
|---|---|---|---|---|---|---|
| 3 | Trifirò et al. 2007, 2010 | Subjects age 65 years or older who were taking an antipsychotic drug Subjects were identified via the Dutch Integrated Primary Care Information database as having incident community-acquired pneumonia. *Design:* population-based, nested case-control study *Location:* Netherlands *Funding:* none | 258 case subjects with incident pneumonia were matched to 1,686 control subjects on the basis of age, sex, and date of onset | 1996–2006 | Sixty-five (25%) of the case subjects died in 30 days with death attributable to pneumonia. Using conditional logistic regression, the study authors found that current use of either an FGA (OR=1.76; CI: 1.22, 2.53) or SGA (OR=2.61; 95% CI: 1.48, 4.61) was associated with a dose-dependent increase in the risk for pneumonia compared with past use of antipsychotic drugs. Current use of SGAs was not associated with an increase in odds ratio of pneumonia relative to FGAs (1.48; 95% CI: 0.84, 2.60). Only SGAs were associated with an increase in the risk for fatal pneumonia (OR=5.97; CI: 1.49, 23.98). | 0 |

*Note.* 1=randomized controlled trial; 2=systematic review/meta-analysis; 3=observational; A=from AHRQ review.
*Cited with other outcome.
AHRQ=Agency for Healthcare Research and Quality; CI=confidence interval; FGA=first-generation antipsychotic; IRR=incidence rate ratio; MI=myocardial infarction; RR=rate ratio; SGA=second-generation antipsychotic; VTE=venous thromboembolism.

## Quality of the Body of Research Evidence for Harm Related to Pulmonary Events

*Risk of bias:* **Moderate**—Studies include two placebo-controlled RCTs with small numbers of pulmonary events in each trial condition and six observational studies that are of low quality due to the lack of randomization, potential confounds of administrative database studies, and the lack of restriction of some studies to individuals with a presumptive diagnosis of dementia.

*Consistency:* **Inconsistent**—Findings are variable in the small number of available studies. Only one study was available for VTE, so no assessment of consistency was possible.

*Directness:* **Direct**—Studies measure rates of pneumonia and rates of VTE, which are directly related to the PICOTS question on effects. An increased risk of VTE could indirectly affect rates of pulmonary embolism and associated pulmonary dysfunction.

*Precision:* **Imprecise**—Confidence intervals for the odds ratios in the observational studies are large for pneumonia and for VTE.

*Applicability:* Several of the observational studies include older individuals without specifying a diagnosis. Observational studies include subjects from Canada, Australia, Germany, and the Netherlands. The observational studies include a mix of nursing home and community-based subjects.

*Dose-response relationship:* **Unknown**—This was not assessed in the reported studies.

*Magnitude of effect:* **Weak effect**—The effect size is small in the majority of the studies; studies with a higher odds ratio also have very wide confidence intervals, and so interpretation is difficult. For the two placebo-controlled studies, results were not significant for individual medications.

*Confounding factors:* **Present**—The data from the observational studies have a number of potentially confounding factors. Because no information is available on co-occurring medical conditions in individuals receiving antipsychotic medications, these individuals may have been at greater risk of adverse outcomes independent of their use of antipsychotic medication. They also may have had a greater severity of dementia at the time of treatment, which could also affect the development of pneumonia (due to swallowing impairments) and VTE (due to immobility).

*Publication bias:* **Not suspected**—There is no specific evidence to suggest selection bias.

*Overall strength of evidence:* **Low**.

## Neurological Side Effects: Cognitive Changes
### Overview and Quality of Individual Studies

The authors of the 2011 AHRQ report (Maglione et al. 2011) noted that in six head-to-head trials of SGAs, patients receiving olanzapine had higher likelihoods of neurological symptoms such as confusion, headaches, and dizziness compared with those receiving risperidone, whereas aripiprazole and quetiapine did not differ from placebo in the frequency of these effects. The CATIE-AD trial showed cognitive decline with olanzapine, quetiapine, or risperidone (Vigen et al. 2011).

Of the two observational trials identified subsequent to the AHRQ report, one study found a slower decline in cognition with antipsychotic treatment, whereas the other study showed a more rapid decline. There is also a potential for significant confounds in terms of dementia severity and neuropsychiatric symptoms that led to initiation of antipsychotic treatment.

**TABLE A–34. Overview of studies examining risk of cognitive changes with antipsychotics**

| Study type | Study | Subject/Method/Design/Location | N | Duration | Outcomes/Results | Rating of quality of evidence |
|---|---|---|---|---|---|---|
| 3 | Dutcher et al. 2014 | Older nursing home residents with newly diagnosed Alzheimer's disease or related dementias Subjects were identified based on Medicare enrollment and claims data linked to the Minimum Dataset 2.0. *Design:* prospective cohort study *Location:* United States | 18,950 subjects with a mean age of 83.6 years; 76% of the sample subjects were female. At baseline, 15% were taking antidementia medications, 40% antidepressants, 13% antipsychotics, and 3% mood stabilizers. | 2007–2008 | Using marginal structural models to account for time-dependent confounding, the study authors found that antipsychotic use was associated with a slower decline in cognition (slope difference: −0.11 points/year on the CPS, 99% CI: −0.17, −0.06), with more rapid declines observed in females. However, the magnitude of these changes was not noted to be clinically significant, although it was statistically significant. | 0 |
| 3 | Rosenberg et al. 2012 | Community-ascertained case patients from the Cache County Dementia Progression Study who had incident Alzheimer's disease *Design:* prospective cohort *Location:* United States | 230 case subjects | Mean follow-up 3.7 years | At baseline, psychotropic medication use was associated with greater severity of dementia, and poorer medical status was associated with use of psychotropic medications (e.g., antidepressants, antipsychotics, benzodiazepines). Mixed-effects models showed that a higher proportion of observed time of medication exposure was associated with a more rapid decline in MMSE for all medication classes, including antipsychotic agents. In terms of FGAs, a higher proportion of observed time of medication exposure was associated with a more rapid increase in CDR Sum of Boxes and NPI total score. | 0 |

| Study type | Study | Subject/Method/Design/Location | N | Duration | Outcomes/Results | Rating of quality of evidence |
|---|---|---|---|---|---|---|
| 1 | Vigen et al. 2011 | Ambulatory outpatients living at home or in an assisted-living facility whose symptoms met DSM-IV criteria for dementia of the Alzheimer's type or NINCDS/ADRDA criteria for probable Alzheimer's disease and who had delusions, hallucinations, agitation, or aggression nearly every day over the previous week or intermittently over 4 weeks<br>*Design:* multiphase, multisite double-blind, randomized study. After initial treatment phase, subsequent phases and randomization were dependent on response to initial treatment assignment. Patients could be taking cholinesterase inhibitor medication but not antidepressants or anticonvulsants for mood disorder.<br>*Location:* United States | 421 patients were randomly assigned in a double-blind fashion to receive olanzapine, quetiapine, risperidone, or placebo (randomized allocation 2:2:2:3). 342 subjects had at least one follow-up cognitive measure at 12 weeks, 320 at 24 weeks, and 307 at 36 weeks. Sample patients were 46% male, with a mean age of 77.6 years and a mean of 12.3 years of education ; 64% were taking cholinesterase inhibitors. | 36 weeks | Significant declines occurred in multiple cognitive measures, including the MMSE ($P=0.004$), BPRS Cognitive subscale ($P=0.05$), and a cognitive summary score summarizing change on 18 cognitive tests ($P=0.004$). Declines were linear and significant over time (e.g., 2.4-point decrease in MMSE and a 4.4-point decrease in ADAS-Cog over 36 weeks) without effects of baseline MMSE, baseline BPRS score, or size of the study site. Patients taking an SGA for at least 2 weeks showed a greater rate of decline in cognitive function than those receiving placebo, although these declines were not statistically significant for all measures. | 1 |

*Note.* 1=randomized controlled trial; 2=systematic review/meta-analysis; 3=observational; A=from AHRQ review. ADAS-Cog=Alzheimer's Disease Assessment Scale—Cognitive Behavior; AHRQ=Agency for Healthcare Research and Quality; BPRS=Brief Psychiatric Rating Scale; CATIE-AD= Clinical Antipsychotic Trials of Intervention Effectiveness for Alzheimer's Disease; CDR=Clinical Dementia Rating; CI=confidence interval; CPS=Cognitive Performance Scale; FGA=first-generation antipsychotic; MMSE=Mini-Mental State Exam; NINCDS/ADRDA=National Institute of Neurological Disorders and Stroke–Alzheimer's Disease and Related Disorders Association ; NPI=Neuropsychiatric Inventory; SGA=second-generation antipsychotic.

## Quality of the Body of Research Evidence for Harm Related to Cognitive Changes

*Risk of bias:* **Moderate**—Studies include placebo-controlled RCTs that were designed to test efficacy of SGAs in BPSD; neurological changes (including cognition) were not a primary outcome of these trials. Data are also available from the CATIE-AD study and two observational studies. However, the latter two studies are of low quality due to the lack of randomization.

*Consistency:* **Inconsistent**—The studies vary in their findings, with some showing slower cognitive decline and others showing more rapid decline in cognition.

*Directness:* **Indirect**—Studies measure scores on cognitive batteries, but the effect of the antipsychotic medication is not readily distinguishable from the effects of the underlying dementia.

*Applicability:* The included studies primarily involve individuals with dementia. The doses of antipsychotic that were used in the randomized studies are consistent with usual practice. The CATIE-AD trial and the observational studies include subjects from the United States, with some community-based subjects and some subjects who resided in nursing facilities. Randomized trials typically exclude individuals with significant co-occurring medical or psychiatric conditions as well as individuals who require urgent intervention before consent could be obtained, and this may influence the estimation of possible harms in broader groups of patients. For most of the observational studies, information about antipsychotic doses, co-occurring conditions, concomitant medications, and other factors that may influence applicability is unknown.

*Dose-response relationship:* **Unknown**—This was not assessed in the reported studies.

*Magnitude of effect:* **Weak effect**—The effect size is very small and not deemed to be clinically significant in one of the studies.

*Confounding factors:* **Present**—The data from the observational studies have a number of potentially confounding factors. Because no information is available on co-occurring medical conditions in individuals receiving antipsychotic medications, these individuals may have been at greater risk of adverse outcomes independent of their use of antipsychotic medication. They also may have had a greater severity of dementia at the time of treatment, which could also influence subsequent changes in cognition.

*Publication bias:* **Not suspected**—There is no specific evidence to suggest selection bias.
*Overall strength of evidence:* **Low**.

## Sedation and Fatigue

### Overview and Quality of Individual Studies

The authors of the AHRQ review (Maglione et al. 2011) reported that aripiprazole, olanzapine, quetiapine, and risperidone were associated with sedation and increased fatigue. Data on haloperidol and FGAs were not reported. Taken together, the results of placebo-controlled trials showed sedation in 19.5% (622/3,190) subjects treated with an SGA as compared with 8.0% (167/2,089) of subjects receiving placebo. For fatigue, the corresponding proportions were 7.6% (128/1,692) and 1.7% (19/1,088), respectively.

**Pooled data on sedation and fatigue from the 2011 AHRQ review**

| Adverse effect | Drug | Number of studies | Drug (adverse events/ sample size) | Placebo (adverse events/ sample size) | OR | (95% CI) | NNH |
|---|---|---|---|---|---|---|---|
| Fatigue | Aripiprazole | 3 | 47/600 | 11/272 | 2.44 | (1.19, 5.43) | 22 |
| Fatigue | Olanzapine | 3 | 36/482 | 9/326 | 2.37 | (1.08, 5.75) | 34 |
| Fatigue | Quetiapine | 2 | 25/335 | 5/234 | 2.92 | (1.03, 10.26) | 34 |
| Fatigue | Risperidone | 2 | 20/281 | 4/236 | 3.56 | (1.13, 14.96) | 34 |
| Sedation | Aripiprazole | 4 | 116/706 | 22/374 | 2.62 | (1.57, 4.54) | 16 |
| Sedation | Olanzapine | 5 | 158/778 | 25/440 | 4.58 | (2.87, 7.55) | 9 |
| Sedation | Quetiapine | 4 | 84/446 | 18/353 | 5.16 | (2.93, 9.51) | 8 |
| Sedation | Risperidone | 6 | 265/1,260 | 102/922 | 2.33 | (1.79, 3.05) | 10 |

*Note.* AHRQ=Agency for Healthcare Research and Quality; CI=confidence interval; NNH=number needed to harm; OR=odds ratio.
*Source.* Adapted from Maglione et al. 2011.

In the CATIE-AD trial (Schneider et al. 2006), rates of sedation with olanzapine, quetiapine, and risperidone were 24%, 22%, and 15%, respectively, as compared with 5% for placebo ($P<0.001$).

## Quality of the Body of Research Evidence for Harm Related to Sedation and Fatigue

*Risk of bias:* **Low**—Studies include placebo-controlled RCTs with a reasonable number of individuals in each sample condition who experienced sedation or fatigue.

*Consistency:* **Consistent**—Each of the SGAs that were assessed showed a statistically significant increase in sedation and in fatigue relative to placebo.

*Directness:* **Direct**—Studies measure rates of sedation and fatigue, which are directly related to the PICOTS question on adverse effects.

*Precision:* **Precise**—Confidence intervals for the odds ratios from the pooled randomized data are small to moderate, and none of the confidence intervals include negative values.

*Applicability:* The included studies all involve individuals with dementia. The doses of antipsychotic that were used in the randomized studies are consistent with usual practice. The randomized and observational studies include subjects from multiple countries and settings.

*Dose-response relationship:* **Unknown**—This was not reported in the analysis.

*Magnitude of effect:* **Moderate effect**—The effect size is moderate, with a two- to fivefold increase in treated subjects relative to untreated subjects, and with some variability by medication.

*Confounding factors:* **Present**—Many of the studies permit use of lorazepam or other "rescue" medications for significant agitation, which is not taken into account in the analysis.

*Publication bias:* **Not suspected**—There is no specific evidence to suggest selection bias.

*Overall strength of evidence:* **Moderate**.

# Extrapyramidal Symptoms

## Overview and Quality of Individual Studies

Moderate strength of evidence suggested that olanzapine and risperidone were associated with an increase in extrapyramidal signs or extrapyramidal symptoms (EPS) relative to placebo. On the basis of data pooled from four placebo-controlled trials of aripiprazole, five of risperidone, and three of quetiapine, risperidone was prone to an increase in EPS, compared with placebo, but aripiprazole and quetiapine were not. In one trial of olanzapine, the olanzapine group was more likely to report EPS than was the placebo group. The authors of the 2011 AHRQ review (Maglione et al. 2011) reported no effect of olanzapine, quetiapine, or risperidone on the development of tardive dyskinesia (TD), however the clinical trial durations would not have been long enough to identify new-onset TD in a reliable fashion.

TABLE A–36. Pooled data on extrapyramidal symptoms, akathisia, and tardive dyskinesia from the 2011 AHRQ review

| Adverse effect | Drug | Number of studies | Drug (adverse events/ sample size) | Placebo (adverse events/ sample size) | OR | (95% CI) | NNH |
|---|---|---|---|---|---|---|---|
| EPS | Aripiprazole | 4 | 39/706 | 16/374 | 1.29 | (0.68, 2.57) | NC |
| EPS | Olanzapine | 1 | 18/100 | 2/142 | 15.21 | (3.50, 138.55) | 10 |
| EPS | Quetiapine | 3 | 18/355 | 9/254 | 1.15 | (0.46, 3.08) | NC |
| EPS | Risperidone | 5 | 130/1,561 | 31/916 | 3.00 | (1.96, 4.70) | 20 |
| Akathisia | Olanzapine | 1 | 1/100 | 0/142 | inf+ | (0.04, inf+) | NC |
| Akathisia | Quetiapine | 2 | 1/114 | 1/162 | 1.23 | (0.02, 98.52) | NC |
| Akathisia | Risperidone | 1 | 0/85 | 0/142 | NC | NC | NC |
| TD | Olanzapine | 1 | 3/100 | 4/142 | 1.07 | (0.15, 6.46) | NC |
| TD | Quetiapine | 1 | 2/94 | 4/142 | 0.75 | (0.07, 5.36) | NC |
| TD | Risperidone | 4 | 4/949 | 14/713 | 0.31 | (0.07, 1.03) | NC |

*Note.* CI=confidence interval; EPS=extrapyramidal symptoms; inf+=infinity; NC=not calculated; NNH=number needed to harm; OR=odds ratio; TD=tardive dyskinesia.
*Source.* Adapted from Maglione et al. 2011.

In the CATIE-AD trial, subjects taking risperidone or olanzapine were more likely to develop EPS than those treated with quetiapine or placebo. In the two observational studies identified since the AHRQ report, risperidone had a lower risk of EPS than FGAs. In the second study, risperidone, olanzapine, and quetiapine had comparable risk of EPS at usual clinical doses. An additional observational study showed comparable rates for tardive dyskinesia with FGAs as compared with SGAs.

| Study type | Study | Subject/Method/ Design/Location | *N* | Duration | Outcomes/Results | Rating of quality of evidence |
|---|---|---|---|---|---|---|
| 3 | Lee et al. 2005 | Subjects age 66 years or older with a diagnosis of dementia who were identified via the Ontario Drug Benefits database as having initiated treatment with an antipsychotic agent <br> *Design:* observational-retrospective cohort <br> *Location:* Ontario, Canada <br> *Funding:* Canadian Institutes of Health Research | 21,835 subjects; 12,045 of the subjects initiated treatment with an FGA, and 9,790 initiated treatment with an SGA | April 1, 1997– March 31, 2001 | TD or other movement disorder was documented as a diagnosis for 3.0% of subjects prescribed an FGA and 3.5% of subjects prescribed an SGA. Rates of TD or other drug-induced movement disorder with FGAs and SGAs were 5.24 and 5.19 cases per 100 person-years for treatment, respectively. Using Cox proportional hazards analysis, the study authors found that the relative risk of a drug-induced movement disorder did not differ for SGAs as compared with FGAs (relative risk=0.99; 95% CI: 0.86, 1.15). | 0 |
| 3 | Marras et al. 2012 | Subjects with dementia who were newly prescribed quetiapine, olanzapine, or risperidone <br> Subjects were identified with administrative database information. <br> *Design:* observational-retrospective cohort <br> *Location:* Ontario Canada | 51,878 subjects | 2002–2010 | From 15,939 person-years of observation, 421 patients developed parkinsonism. <br> With low-dose risperidone as the reference group, the adjusted hazard ratios for developing parkinsonism were 0.49 (95% CI: 0.07, 3.53) for low-dose olanzapine and 1.18 (95% CI: 0.84, 1.66) for low-dose quetiapine. <br> When comparisons were made across drugs within the most commonly prescribed dose ranges, the incidence of parkinsonism was higher in the medium-dose olanzapine group compared with the low-dose risperidone group (HR=1.66; 95% CI: 0.23, 2.23). <br> Adjusted hazard ratio for developing parkinsonism for men (compared with women) was 2.29 (95% CI: 1.88, 2.79). | 0 |

**TABLE A–37.** Overview of studies examining risk of extrapyramidal side effects with antipsychotics *(continued)*

| Study type | Study | Subject/Method/Design/Location | N | Duration | Outcomes/Results | Rating of quality of evidence |
|---|---|---|---|---|---|---|
| 1 | Schneider et al. 2006* | Subjects with Alzheimer's disease or probable Alzheimer's disease (MMSE scores 5–26), ambulatory and residing at home or in assisted living facilities, with moderate or greater levels of psychosis, aggression, or agitation<br>*Interventions:* Placebo vs. masked, flexibly dosed olanzapine (mean dose: 5.5 mg/day), quetiapine (mean dose: 56.5 mg/day), or risperidone (mean dose: 1.0 mg/day)<br>Stable doses of cholinesterase inhibitor were permitted.<br>*Design:* Multicenter, federally funded CATIE-AD trial—Phase 1 | 421 subjects randomly assigned to treatment group, with 142 receiving placebo, 100 receiving olanzapine, 94 receiving quetiapine, and 85 receiving risperidone | Median duration on Phase 1 treatment was 7.1 weeks; clinical outcomes assessed for those who continued to take an antipsychotic at 12 weeks | Subjects treated with olanzapine and risperidone had higher rates of extrapyramidal signs (12% in each group) compared with subjects treated with quetiapine or receiving placebo (2% and 1%, respectively). Similar findings were noted in terms of SAS ratings of greater than 1, which were more frequent with olanzapine (14%) and risperidone (11%) than with placebo (2%). | 1 |
| 3 | Vasilyeva et al. 2013 | Residents of Manitoba, Canada age 65 years or older who had an antipsychotic medication dispensed for the first time during the study period<br>Subjects were identified via Manitoba's Department of Health administrative databases.<br>*Design:* observational-retrospective cohort, population-based sample<br>*Location:* Manitoba, Canada | 8,885 persons in the sample were identified as receiving an antipsychotic medication (accounting for values of 4.3% of males and 6.0% of females), with 4,242 persons in the group who received an FGA and 4,643 in the group who received risperidone | April 1, 2000–March 31, 2007 | Using Cox proportional hazards models to determine the risk of extrapyramidal symptoms in new users of risperidone compared with new users of FGAs, the study authors found that risperidone use was associated with a lower risk of EPS compared with FGAs at 30, 60, 90, and 180 days (adjusted HR=0.38 [95% CI: 0.22, 0.67], 0.45 [95% CI: 0.28, 0.73], 0.50 [95% CI: 0.33, 0.77], 0.65 [95% CI: 0.45, 0.94], respectively) after controlling for potential confounders (demographics, comorbidity, and medication use). At 360 days, the strength of the association had weakened, with an adjusted HR of 0.75 (95% CI: 0.54, 1.05). | 0 |

*Note.* 1=randomized controlled trial; 2=systematic review/meta-analysis; 3=observational; A=from AHRQ review.
*Cited with other outcome.
ADAS-Cog=Alzheimer's Disease Assessment Scale—Cognitive Behavior; AHRQ=Agency for Healthcare Research and Quality; CATIE-AD= Clinical Antipsychotic Trials of Intervention Effectiveness for Alzheimer's Disease; CI=confidence interval; FGA=first-generation antipsychotic; HR=hazard ratio; MMSE=Mini-Mental State Exam; SAS=Simpson-Angus Scale; TD=tardive dyskinesia.

## Quality of the Body of Research Evidence for Harm Related to Extrapyramidal Side Effects

*Risk of bias:* **Low**—Studies include placebo-controlled RCTs, including the CATIE-AD trial. Data from observational studies are of lower quality but include a large sample size.

*Consistency:* **Consistent**—Pooled data from randomized placebo-controlled trials, data from the CATIE-AD study, and findings from observational studies all support an increased likelihood of EPS in individuals with dementia who are treated with antipsychotic medication.

*Directness:* **Direct**—Studies measure rates of EPS, which are directly related to the PICOTS question on adverse effects.

*Precision:* **Precise**—Confidence intervals for the odds ratios from the pooled randomized data are narrow with the exception of those for olanzapine, for which only one trial had available results.

*Applicability:* The included studies involve individuals with dementia, with the exception of two of the observational studies that also included other individuals older than 65 who were treated with a newly dispensed antipsychotic medication. The doses of antipsychotic that were used in the randomized studies are consistent with usual practice. The CATIE-AD study and observational studies include subjects from the United States and Canada. It is not clear how many of the studies included nursing facility patients, which may limit applicability. Randomized trials typically exclude individuals with significant co-occurring medical or psychiatric conditions as well as individuals who require urgent intervention before consent could be obtained, and this may influence the estimation of possible harms in broader groups of patients.

*Dose-response relationship:* **Unknown**—This was not assessed in the reported studies.

*Magnitude of effect:* **Moderate effect**—The effect size is small to moderate depending on the specific medication being used.

*Confounding factors:* **Absent**—The majority of the available data are from placebo-controlled trials without apparent confounding factors.

*Publication bias:* **Not suspected**—There is no specific evidence to suggest selection bias.
*Overall strength of evidence:* **Moderate**.

## Falls and Hip Fractures

### Overview and Quality of Individual Studies

In the 2011 AHRQ report (Maglione et al. 2011), falls were not assessed per se, but risperidone and olanzapine had a statistically increased likelihood of problems with gait. Gait issues with aripiprazole and quetiapine did not differ from those with placebo, but confidence intervals were extremely large.

| Adverse effect | Drug | Number of studies | Drug (adverse events/ sample size) | Placebo (adverse events/ sample size) | OR | (95% CI) | NNH |
|---|---|---|---|---|---|---|---|
| Gait issues | Aripiprazole | 1 | 16/366 | 1/121 | 5.47 | (0.83, 231.93) | NC |
| Gait issues | Olanzapine | 4 | 79/641 | 15/373 | 2.75 | (1.52, 5.29) | 21 |
| Gait issues | Quetiapine | 3 | 18/426 | 6/333 | 2.36 | (0.85, 7.59) | NC |
| Gait issues | Risperidone | 3 | 32/448 | 8/406 | 3.04 | (1.32, 7.84) | 33 |

*Note.* CI=confidence interval; NC=not calculated; NNH=number needed to harm; OR=odds ratio.
*Source.* Adapted from Maglione et al. 2011.

In the CATIE-AD trial, rates of falls (including those with injury or fracture) did not differ for the SGAs as compared with placebo. In observational studies, one study found increased fall rates with antipsychotic treatment, with risk that was greater at higher doses of medication. Use of other psychotropic medications also increased risk of falls, particularly when multiple psychotropic agents were used concomitantly. Three additional observational studies examined rates of hip fracture with antipsychotic treatment in individuals over 65 years of age or nursing home residents. Only one of these studies was limited to individuals with dementia. Two of the studies showed an increased risk of hip fracture following initiation of an antipsychotic. However, one study showed an increased rate of hip fractures in the period prior to antipsychotic initiation, suggesting that agitation or psychosis may predispose to falls and hip fractures or that patients became delirious and required antipsychotic medication following a hip fracture. In two studies, use of FGAs was associated with a greater risk of hip fracture than use of SGAs. When the results are taken together, however, there appears to be an increase in the risk of falls and hip fractures of approximately 1.5- to 2.5-fold in association with antipsychotic treatment.

| Study type | Study | Subject/Method/ Design/Location | N | Duration | Outcomes/Results | Rating of quality of evidence |
|---|---|---|---|---|---|---|
| 3A | Huybrechts et al. 2011* | Nursing home residents age 65 years or older who had treatment with psychotropics initiated after admission<br>*Design:* retrospective population-based cohort<br>*Location:* British Columbia | 10,900 subjects; an SGA was begun in 1,942, an FGA in 1,902, an antidepressant in 2,169, and a benzodiazepine in 4,887 | 1996–2006 | Using proportional hazards models with propensity-score adjustments, the study authors found that users of FGAs had an increased risk of death (RR=1.47, 95% CI: 1.14, 1.91), and an increased risk of femur fracture within 180 days after treatment initiation (RR=1.61, 95% CI: 1.03, 2.51), as compared with users of SGAs. Users of benzodiazepines also had a higher risk of death (RR=1.28, 95% CI: 1.04, 1.58) compared with users of SGAs. There was no difference observed in the risk of heart failure or pneumonia in individuals receiving FGAs, as compared with SGAs (RR=1.03 [95% CI: 0.62, 1.69] and 0.91 [95% CI: 0.41, 2.01], respectively). Using subgroup adjusted propensity scores, the study authors found that individuals who started taking an FGA (as compared with users of an SGA) had an increased risk of mortality, with an RR of 1.37 (95% CI: 0.96, 1.95) for individuals with dementia and 1.61 (95% CI: 1.10, 2.36) for individuals without dementia. Among individuals with no history of antipsychotic treatment, the corresponding RR was 1.33 (95% CI: 0.99, 1.77) as compared with users of an SGA. | 0 |

| Study type | Study | Subject/Method/ Design/Location | N | Duration | Outcomes/Results | Rating of quality of evidence |
|---|---|---|---|---|---|---|
| 3 | Jalbert et al. 2010 | Subjects age 65 years or older with a diagnosis of dementia and no record of a previous hip fracture; long-stay Medicaid-eligible residents living in one of 586 nursing homes in California, Florida, Illinois, New York, or Ohio Subjects were identified via Medicaid claims data. Excluded were individuals who were receiving hospice care, comatose, bedfast, paralyzed, or in a wheelchair. *Design:* nested case-control study *Location:* United States *Funding:* not explicitly stated | 69,027 individuals in total database; 764 of these individuals had experienced a hip fracture and were matched with up to 5 randomly selected controls (N=3,582) | 2001–2002 | Current use of an antipsychotic was associated with a small increase in the risk of hospitalization for hip fracture (adjusted OR=1.26; 95% CI: 1.05, 1.52). Risk of hip fracture was slightly higher for new users of antipsychotics (adjusted OR=1.33; 95% CI: 0.95, 1.88) than for ongoing users (adjusted OR=1.21; 95% CI: 0.99, 1.47). For current users of FGAs, risk was higher (adjusted OR=1.44; 95% CI: 0.84, 2.47) than for SGAs (adjusted OR=1.27; 95% CI: 1.05, 1.54). Corresponding odds ratios for current users of specific SGAs were olanzapine (adjusted OR=1.41; 95% CI: 1.08, 1.84), risperidone (adjusted OR=1.35; 95% CI: 1.07, 1.70), and quetiapine (adjusted OR=1.30; 95% CI: 0.86, 1.96). Sample sizes were insufficient to calculate adjusted ORs for the other specific antipsychotics. Case and control subjects were similar on most measures, but case subjects had a greater frequency and severity of behavioral and psychological symptoms of dementia. | 0 |

| Study type | Study | Subject/Method/Design/Location | N | Duration | Outcomes/Results | Rating of quality of evidence |
|---|---|---|---|---|---|---|
| 3 | Pratt et al. 2011 | Subjects over 65 years of age who were exposed to antipsychotic medication<br>Subjects were identified via Australian Government Department of Veterans' Affairs Health Care Claims Database.<br>*Design:* observational-retrospective cohort<br>*Location:* Australia<br>*Funding:* Australian Government | 8,235 subjects had had at least one hospitalization for hip fracture; 494 of these subjects had started receiving an FGA and 1,091 had started receiving an SGA. 13,324 had had at least one hospitalization for pneumonia; 807 of these subjects had started receiving an FGA and 1,107 had started receiving an SGA during the study period. | 2005–2008; median follow-up: 3.3–4.0 years | Using a self-controlled case-series design, the study authors found a significantly increased risk of hip fracture with use of an FGA during all postexposure risk periods beginning at 1 week of exposure. Risk remained significantly increased with more than 12 weeks of continuous exposure (IRR=2.19; 95% CI: 1.62, 2.95). After initiation of SGAs, the risk of hip fracture was highest in the first week (IRR=2.17; 95% CI: 1.54, 3.06) and then declined but remained significantly raised with more than 12 weeks of continuous exposure (IRR=1.43; 95% CI: 1.23, 1.66). The study also found a significantly increased risk of hospitalization for hip fracture up to 16 weeks prior to antipsychotic initiation. | 0 |

| Study type | Study | Subject/Method/Design/Location | N | Duration | Outcomes/Results | Rating of quality of evidence |
|---|---|---|---|---|---|---|
| 1 | Schneider et al. 2006* | Subjects with Alzheimer's disease or probable Alzheimer's disease (MMSE scores 5–26), ambulatory and residing at home or in assisted living facilities, with moderate or greater levels of psychosis, aggression, or agitation *Interventions:* placebo vs. masked, flexibly dosed olanzapine (mean dose: 5.5 mg/day), quetiapine (mean dose: 56.5 mg/day), or risperidone (mean dose: 1.0 mg/day) Stable doses of cholinesterase inhibitor were permitted. *Design:* multicenter, federally funded CATIE-AD trial—Phase 1 | 421 subjects randomly assigned to treatment group, with 142 receiving placebo, 100 receiving olanzapine, 94 receiving quetiapine, and 85 receiving risperidone | Median duration on Phase 1 treatment was 7.1 weeks; clinical outcomes assessed for those who were continuing to take antipsychotic at 12 weeks | Falls, injuries, and fractures were reported together. No significant differences were found between subjects treated with SGAs and those receiving placebo with rates of 17% for olanzapine, 7% for quetiapine, and 12% for risperidone as compared with a rate of 15% for placebo. | 1 |

| Study type | Study | Subject/Method/ Design/Location | N | Duration | Outcomes/Results | Rating of quality of evidence |
|---|---|---|---|---|---|---|
| 3 | Sterke et al. 2012 | Nursing home residents with dementia who had data on drug use abstracted from a prescription database and falls identified using a standardized incident report system *Design:* observational-retrospective cohort *Location:* Netherlands | 248 subjects, accounting for 85,074 person-days, with an antipsychotic being used in 45.4% of these person-days | January 1, 2006– January 1, 2008 | Fall risk was increased with the use of antipsychotics (HR=1.53; 95% CI: 1.17, 2.00). Fall risk was also increased with age (HR=1.05; 95% CI: 1.02, 1.08) and with use of anxiolytics (1.60; 95% CI: 1.19, 2.16), hypnotics and sedatives (1.50; 95% CI: 1.04, 2.16), and antidepressants (2.28; 95% CI: 1.58, 3.29). There was a significant dose-response relationship between fall risk and use of antipsychotics (HR=2.78; 95% CI: 1.49, 5.17). Also associated with a significant dose-response relationship and an increased risk of falls were anxiolytics (1.60; 95% CI: 1.20, 2.14), hypnotics and sedatives (2.58; 95% CI: 1.42, 4.68), and antidepressants (2.84; 95% CI: 1.93, 4.16). For antipsychotics, fall risk was increased even at low doses (25% of the average dosage of a drug taken by adults for the main indication as indicated by the World Health Organization); fall risk increased further with dose increments and with combinations of psychotropics. | 0 |

*Note.* 1=randomized controlled trial; 2=systematic review/meta-analysis; 3=observational; A=from AHRQ review. *Cited with other outcome.
AHRQ=Agency for Healthcare Research and Quality; CATIE-AD= Clinical Antipsychotic Trials of Intervention Effectiveness for Alzheimer's Disease; CI=confidence interval; FGA=first-generation antipsychotic; HR=hazard ratio; IRR=incidence rate ratio; MMSE=Mini-Mental State Exam; RR=rate ratio; SGA=second-generation antipsychotic.

## Quality of the Body of Research Evidence for Harm Related to Falls and Hip Fractures

*Risk of bias:* **Moderate**—Placebo-controlled RCTs describe gait difficulties with SGAs but do not consistently report rates of falls, with the exception of the CATIE-AD study. Observational studies are of low quality due to the lack of randomization, potential confounds of administrative database studies, and the lack of restriction of some studies to individuals with a presumptive diagnosis of dementia.

*Consistency:* **Inconsistent**—Observational studies are consistent in suggesting an increased risk of falls and hip fracture with antipsychotic medications; however, the CATIE-AD trial did not report any differences in fall, injury, or fracture rates relative to placebo.

*Directness:* **Direct**—Studies measure rates of falls and hip fractures, which are directly related to the PICOTS question on adverse effects.

*Precision:* **Imprecise**—Confidence intervals for the odds ratios from observational studies are relatively narrow, but those from the CATIE-AD study overlap the origin.

*Applicability:* The included studies involve individuals with dementia, although some of the administrative database studies included older individuals without specifying a diagnosis. The doses of antipsychotic that were used in the randomized studies are consistent with usual practice. The observational studies include subjects from around the world, including the United States, Canada, Australia, and the Netherlands. The studies include nursing facility patients as well as community dwelling subjects. Randomized trials typically exclude individuals with significant co-occurring medical or psychiatric conditions as well as individuals who require urgent intervention before consent could be obtained, and this may influence the estimation of possible harms in broader groups of patients. Information about antipsychotic doses, co-occurring conditions, concomitant medications, and other factors that may influence applicability was present in some of the studies and enhances the applicability of the findings.

*Dose-response relationship:* **Present**—In at least one study, an increase in risk was present with an increasing dose of medication.

*Magnitude of effect:* **Weak effect**—The effect size is small in the observational studies and nonexistent in the CATIE-AD trial.

*Confounding factors:* **Present**—The data from the observational studies have a number of potentially confounding factors. Individuals in these studies may have been at greater risk of adverse outcomes independent of their use of antipsychotic medication. (The finding in one study of an increase in risk before initiation of antipsychotic medication is consistent with such a hypothesis.) They also may have had a greater severity of dementia at the time of treatment, which could also impact adverse outcomes.

*Publication bias:* **Not suspected**—There is no specific evidence to suggest selection bias.

*Overall strength of evidence:* **Low**.

## Endocrine Adverse Events

### Overview and Quality of Individual Studies

The authors of the 2011 AHRQ review (Maglione et al. 2011) noted that there was only one placebo-controlled RCT in patients with dementia that reported adverse endocrine outcomes. No difference in diabetes onset or prolactin measures was found between patients receiving risperidone and those receiving placebo, but the number of incident cases was small in all groups. In the CATIE-AD study, no difference was found between changes in glucose and the use of an SGA as compared with placebo. Prolactin levels were significantly increased only in the group that received risperidone (Schneider et al. 2006).

Of two observational studies, one found no increase in diabetic risk for patients treated with olanzapine as compared with other antipsychotic comparators or placebo. The other observational study reported that the use or duration of use of SGAs was not associated with diabetes onset compared with the nonuse of antipsychotics. In contrast, FGA treatment was associated with diabetes onset, particularly when treatment duration was less than 30 days. An additional administrative database study in a sample of older individuals found an increase in hyperglycemic events in users of FGAs and SGAs.

**Overview of studies examining risk of endocrine adverse events with antipsychotics**

| Study type | Study | Subject/Method/Design/Location | N | Duration | Outcomes/Results | Rating of quality of evidence |
|---|---|---|---|---|---|---|
| 3 | Jalbert et al. 2011 | Nursing home residents age 65 years or older with dementia and no record of diabetes within 90 days of nursing home admission; long-stay Medicaid-eligible residents living in nursing homes in California, Florida, Illinois, New York, and Ohio. Cases of incident diabetes were identified via MDS assessments and Medicaid claims, medication use was ascertained from Medicaid pharmacy files, and resident characteristics were obtained from MDS assessments. *Interventions:* FGAs or SGAs vs. antipsychotic nonusers. *Design:* observational-case control. *Location:* United States. *Funding:* unfunded study | 29,203 people; 762 incident cases of diabetes identified and up to 5 control cases randomly selected, with case and control subjects matched on nursing home and quarter of MDS assessment (N=2,646) | Recruited from January 2001 to December 2002 | Relative to nonusers of antipsychotics, use of SGAs was not associated with diabetes onset (adjusted OR=1.03; 95% CI: 0.84, 1.27) and risk of diabetes did not increase with length of time on treatment. FGA treatment was associated with diabetes onset, particularly when treatment duration was less than 30 days (adjusted OR=2.70; 95% CI: 1.57, 4.65). | 0 |
| 3 | Lipscombe et al. 2011 | Subjects over 65 years of age without prior diabetes, who had treatment with an antipsychotic medication initiated. Subjects were identified via a population-based health database; 42% of the sample had dementia. *Design:* nested case control. *Location:* Ontario, Canada. Funding: Canadian Institutes of Health Research | 44,121 subjects; 220 of the subjects had had a hospital visit for hyperglycemia and 2,190 served as matched control subjects | Recruited from April 1, 2002, and March 31, 2006, with an average follow-up duration of 2.2 years | Any current use of antipsychotic, use of an FGA, and use of an SGA were all associated with an increased adjusted odds ratio of hyperglycemia compared with use in the remote past (1.52 [95% CI: 1.07, 2.17], 1.44 [95% CI: 1.01, 2.07], and 2.86 [95% CI: 1.46, 3.59], respectively). | 0 |

| Study type | Study | Subject/Method/ Design/Location | N | Duration | Outcomes/ Results | Rating of quality of evidence |
|---|---|---|---|---|---|---|
| 1A | Micca et al. 2006 | Subjects over 65 years of age, who had been diagnosed with dementia Subjects identified via an olanzapine clinical trial database. *Design:* post hoc analysis of pooled data from clinical trials *Location:* not specified *Funding:* pharmaceutical (Eli Lilly) | 1,398 subjects; 835 of the subjects received olanzapine (mean modal dose across all studies was 4.87 mg/day), 223 received an active comparator (risperidone, haloperidol, or another FGA), and 340 received placebo | Not specified | No statistically significant increase in the risk of treatment-emergent diabetes (HR = 1.36), defined as 2 glucose values over 200 mg/dL after baseline (or 1 value at the final visit), initiation of antidiabetic medication, or clinical diagnosis of diabetes was noted. Other risk factors, such as BMI 25 kg/m$^2$ or having at least 7% weight gain during the study, were also not significant (HR=0.86 and HR=2.26, respectively). | 0 |
| 1 | Zheng et al. 2009* | Subjects with Alzheimer's disease or probable Alzheimer's disease (MMSE scores 5–26), ambulatory and residing at home or in assisted living facilities, with moderate or greater levels of psychosis, aggression, or agitation *Interventions:* Phase 1—placebo vs. masked, flexibly dosed olanzapine (mean dose: 5.5 mg/day), quetiapine (mean dose: 56.5 mg/day), or risperidone (mean dose: 1.0 mg/day); Phase 2—antipsychotic or citalopram; Phase 3— open label Stable doses of cholinesterase inhibitor were permitted. *Design:* multicenter, federally funded CATIE-AD trial—Phase 1 | 421 subjects randomly assigned in Phase 1, with 142 receiving placebo, 100 receiving olanzapine, 94 receiving quetiapine, and 85 receiving risperidone | Median duration on Phase 1 treatment was 7.1 weeks; total trial duration: 36 weeks | No treatment effects were noted for changes in blood pressure, glucose, and triglycerides, but olanzapine was significantly associated with decreases in high-density lipoprotein cholesterol (−0.19 mg/dL/ week) and increased girth (0.07 inches/week) relative to the placebo group. | 1 |

*Note.* 1=randomized controlled trial; 2=systematic review/meta-analysis; 3=observational; A=from AHRQ review.
*Cited with other outcome.
AHRQ–Agency for Healthcare Research and Quality; BMI=body mass index; CATIE-AD– Clinical Antipsychotic Trials of Intervention Effectiveness for Alzheimer's Disease; CI=confidence interval; FGA=first-generation antipsychotic; HR=hazard ratio; MDS=Minimum Data Set; MMSE=Mini-Mental State Exam; OR=odds ratio; SGA=second-generation antipsychotic.

## Quality of the Body of Research Evidence for Harm Related to Endocrine Effects

*Risk of bias:* **Moderate**—With the exception of the CATIE-AD trial, only a small number of placebo-controlled RCTs assessed endocrine effects, and these were not primary study outcomes. Observational studies are of low quality due to the lack of randomization and potential confounds of administrative database studies. One of the studies was an industry sponsored study of pooled post hoc findings, which may also introduce bias.

*Consistency:* **Inconsistent**—One study noted an increased risk of diabetes with FGAs, whereas other studies using SGAs did not find an increase in risk. A third study of older subjects found an increase in hyperglycemia risk for FGAs and SGAs.

*Directness:* **Indirect**—Studies measure glucose levels, lipid levels, and other measures rather than diagnoses of diabetes or metabolic syndrome.

*Precision:* **Imprecise**—Confidence intervals for odds ratios are relatively narrow, but the range of confidence intervals includes negative values in some cases.

*Applicability:* The included studies primarily involve individuals with dementia, although one administrative database study involved older individuals, about 42% of whom had dementia. The doses of antipsychotic that were used in the randomized studies are consistent with usual practice. The studies include U.S. and Canadian patients in nursing facilities and community settings. The observational studies and the CATIE-AD study include subjects with a range of co-occurring conditions, consistent with usual practice.

*Dose-response relationship:* **Unknown**—This was not reported with respect to these parameters.

*Magnitude of effect:* **Weak effect**—The effect size is small when present.

*Confounding factors:* **Present**—The data from the observational studies have a number of potentially confounding factors.

*Publication bias:* **Not suspected**—There is no specific evidence to suggest selection bias.

*Overall strength of evidence:* **Low**.

# Appetite/Weight

## Overview and Quality of Individual Studies

The authors of the AHRQ report (Maglione et al. 2011) found weight gain to be a risk of treatment with antipsychotic medications, although more data are available in younger individuals than in elders with dementia. Pooled data from placebo-controlled trials found that olanzapine and risperidone were statistically associated with increased appetite/weight.

TABLE A–41. Pooled data on weight gain from the 2011 AHRQ review

| Adverse effect | Drug | Number of studies | Drug (adverse events/ sample size) | Placebo (adverse events/ sample size) | OR | (95% CI) | NNH |
|---|---|---|---|---|---|---|---|
| Weight gain | Aripiprazole | 2 | 23/472 | 10/223 | 1.02 | (0.44, 2.49) | NC |
| Weight gain | Olanzapine | 3 | 34/482 | 6/326 | 4.69 | (1.87, 14.14) | 24 |
| Weight gain | Quetiapine | 1 | 5/94 | 4/142 | 1.93 | (0.40, 10.01) | NC |
| Weight gain | Risperidone | 2 | 14/281 | 5/236 | 3.40 | (1.08, 12.75) | 24 |

*Note.* CI=confidence interval; NC=not calculated; NNH=number needed to harm; OR=odds ratio.
*Source.* Adapted from Maglione et al. 2011.

The CATIE-AD head-to-head trial showed some weight gain in patients treated with olanzapine, risperidone, or quetiapine (1.0, 0.4, and 0.7 pounds per month, respectively) compared with a weight loss (0.9 pounds per month) among patients receiving placebo. A cohort study with mostly underweight or normal-weight patients with dementia found a greater chance of gaining weight with olanzapine than with other agents, particularly if the patient's BMI was less than 25 at baseline.

TABLE A–42. Overview of studies examining risk of appetite and weight change with antipsychotics

| Study type | Study | Subject/Method/ Design/Location | N | Duration | Outcomes/Results | Rating of quality of evidence |
|---|---|---|---|---|---|---|
| 3A | Lipkovich et al. 2007 | Individuals over 65 years of age with dementia who were newly pre-scribed olanzapine Subjects identified via an olanzapine clinical trial database. *Design:* observational-retrospective cohort *Location:* United States *Funding:* Eli Lilly | 1,267 subjects | 20 weeks of follow-up | Estimated probability of gaining more than 7% of initial body weight was significantly greater with olanzapine as compared with placebo (*P*<0.001). | 0 |

**Overview of studies examining risk of appetite and weight change with antipsychotics** *(continued)*

| Study type | Study | Subject/Method/ Design/Location | N | Duration | Outcomes/Results | Rating of quality of evidence |
|---|---|---|---|---|---|---|
| 1 | Schneider et al. 2006; Zheng et al. 2009* | Subjects with Alzheimer's disease or probable Alzheimer's disease (MMSE scores 5–26), ambulatory and residing at home or in assisted living facilities, with moderate or greater levels of psychosis, aggression, or agitation<br>*Interventions:* Phase 1—placebo vs. masked, flexibly dosed olanzapine (mean dose: 5.5 mg/day), quetiapine (mean dose: 56.5 mg/day), or risperidone (mean dose: 1.0 mg/day); Phase 2—antipsychotic or citalopram; Phase 3—open label Stable doses of cholinesterase inhibitor were permitted.<br>*Design:* multicenter, federally funded CATIE-AD trial—Phase 1 | 421 subjects randomly assigned in Phase 1, with 142 receiving placebo, 100 receiving olanzapine, 94 receiving quetiapine, and 85 receiving risperidone | Median duration on Phase 1 treatment was 7.1 weeks; total trial duration: 36 weeks | Clinically significant weight gain (i.e., 7% or more of body weight) was seen among patients with antipsychotic use relative to patients who did not use antipsychotics at all time periods during the trial (≤12 weeks: OR=1.56 [95% CI: 0.53, 4.58]; 12 and 24 weeks: OR=2.89 [95% CI: 0.97, 8.64]; >24 weeks OR = 3.38 [95% CI: 1.24, 9.23]). Significant weight gain was noted for women but not for men and for olanzapine and quetiapine but not other study medications. Monthly weight gains ranged from 0.4 to 1.0 lbs as compared with a monthly loss of 0.9 lbs for placebo. | 1 |

*Note.* 1=randomized controlled trial; 2=systematic review/meta-analysis; 3=observational; A=from AHRQ review.
*Cited with other outcome.
AHRQ=Agency for Healthcare Research and Quality; CATIE-AD= Clinical Antipsychotic Trials of Intervention Effectiveness for Alzheimer's Disease; CI=confidence interval; FGA=first-generation antipsychotic; MMSE=Mini-Mental State Exam; OR=odds ratio; SGA=second-generation antipsychotic.

## Quality of the Body of Research Evidence for Harm Related to Appetite and Weight Change

*Risk of bias:* **Low**—Available data are primarily from the CATIE-AD trial, and pooled analyses are from placebo-controlled RCTs.

*Consistency:* **Consistent**—Olanzapine treatment was associated with consistent increases in body weight in several analyses of pooled RCT data as well as in the CATIE-AD trial. Risperidone and quetiapine findings are less consistent but still show increases in weight in some studies.

*Directness:* **Direct**—Studies measure body weight, which is directly related to the PICOTS question on adverse effects.

*Precision:* **Imprecise**—Confidence intervals for the odds ratios from the pooled randomized data are large, and confidence intervals in some studies include negative values.

*Applicability:* The included studies involve individuals with dementia and use doses of antipsychotic that are consistent with usual practice. The study locations include the United States. Studies include community-dwelling subjects, but it is less clear whether nursing facility subjects are included in the pooled RCT analyses.

*Dose-response relationship:* **Unknown**—This was not reported.

*Magnitude of effect:* **Weak effect**—The effect size is small to moderate when an effect is present, but confidence intervals are wide, and this is likely to skew estimates of effect.

*Confounding factors:* **Present**—The data from the observational studies have a number of potentially confounding factors. Because no information is available on co-occurring medical conditions in individuals receiving antipsychotic medications, these individuals may have been at greater risk of adverse outcomes independent of their use of antipsychotic medication. They also may have had a greater severity of dementia at the time of treatment, which could also impact adverse outcomes.

*Publication bias:* **Not suspected**—There is no specific evidence to suggest selection bias.

*Overall strength of evidence:* **Moderate**—The strongest evidence is available for olanzapine, but the evidence is relatively consistent for other SGAs, particularly when known findings in younger subjects are considered.

## Urinary Symptoms

### Overview and Quality of Individual Studies

The authors of the AHRQ report (Maglione et al. 2011) reported that olanzapine, quetiapine, and risperidone were associated with urinary symptoms, compared with placebo, whereas no such association was noted for aripiprazole. One study reported rates of urinary incontinence as an adverse event, whereas in the other reported studies the adverse urinary symptoms consisted of urinary tract infections.

TABLE A–43. **Pooled data on urinary symptoms from the 2011 AHRQ review**

| Adverse effect | Drug | Number of studies | Drug (adverse events/ sample size) | Placebo (adverse events/ sample size) | OR | (95% CI) | NNH |
|---|---|---|---|---|---|---|---|
| Urinary | Aripiprazole | 3 | 115/603 | 44/348 | 1.37 | (0.92, 2.09) | NC |
| Urinary | Olanzapine | 1 | 19/204 | 1/94 | 9.51 | (1.47, 401.07) | 36 |
| Urinary | Quetiapine | 2 | 44/332 | 12/191 | 2.37 | (1.16, 5.15) | 16 |
| Urinary | Risperidone | 4 | 164/1,060 | 71/665 | 1.55 | (1.13, 2.13) | 21 |

*Note.* CI=confidence interval; NNH=number needed to harm; OR=odds ratio.
*Source.* Adapted from Maglione et al. 2011.

## Quality of the Body of Research Evidence for Harm Related to Urinary Symptoms

*Risk of bias:* **Moderate**—Studies include placebo-controlled RCTs, but adverse effects were not a primary outcome of these trials, which were designed to test efficacy.

*Consistency:* **Consistent**—With the exception of quetiapine, pooled data from randomized placebo-controlled trials of SGAs showed statistically increased rates of urinary symptoms as compared with placebo.

*Directness:* **Direct**—Studies measure rates of urinary symptoms, which are directly related to the PICOTS question on adverse effects.

*Precision:* **Imprecise**—Confidence intervals for the odds ratios from the pooled randomized data are relatively large, and the range of confidence intervals includes negative values in one case.

*Applicability:* The included studies involve individuals with dementia. The doses of antipsychotic that were used in the randomized studies are consistent with usual practice. Randomized trials typically exclude individuals with significant co-occurring medical or psychiatric conditions, which may influence the estimation of possible harms in broader groups of patients. Differences may also exist between male and female subjects, and data are not reported in a manner that would allow such distinctions to be made.

*Dose-response relationship:* **Unknown**—This was not assessed in the reported studies.

*Magnitude of effect:* **Weak effect**—The effect size is small for risperidone and quetiapine and not significant for aripiprazole. Olanzapine has a large reported effect, but the extremely large confidence interval makes it difficult to interpret.

*Confounding factors:* **Present**—The data from the studies may have potentially confounding factors. Although these data are from placebo-controlled RCTs, factors such as sex and co-occurring medical conditions may influence urinary symptoms and do not appear to have been accounted for in the analysis.

*Publication bias:* **Not suspected**—There is no specific evidence to suggest selection bias.

*Overall strength of evidence:* **Low.**

# APPENDIX B

# Expert Opinion Survey Data: Results

## Section I: Questions About Appropriate Use

Experts were given the following instructions in terms of providing answers to the survey questions:

> A treatment is appropriate if the expected health benefits (e.g., relief of symptoms, improved functional capacity, improved quality of life, increased life expectancy) exceed expected negative consequences (e.g., adverse effects) by a sufficiently wide margin that the treatment is worth doing, exclusive of cost. The expert opinion about appropriateness is based on both available evidence and their clinical experience.

In the context of these questions, "assessment" is defined as obtaining information about the patient's current symptoms and behavior and past history, including through reports of staff and caregivers. The assessment will typically include the results of a mental status examination by the clinician and may also include readily available laboratory tests, depending on the urgency of the situation.

"Dementia" is a degenerative condition characterized by multiple cognitive deficits that include impairment in memory. It has various etiologies and usually affects older adults. For this survey, the term "dementia" should be understood to be equivalent to the term "major neurocognitive disorder" as defined in DSM-5.

# 1. DANGEROUS AGITATION—Please rate the appropriateness of each treatment for the given clinical circumstance.

**TABLE B–1.** Appropriateness of antipsychotics for the given clinical circumstance (rated using a 1–5 scale, where 1=highly inappropriate, 3=uncertain, and 5=highly appropriate)

**1a.** The agitation is a NEW SYMPTOM. Assessment SUGGESTS a short-term reversible cause of the agitation, such as acute delirium, medication side effects, or environmental causes.

| Appropriateness of use | Aripiprazole (n=203) | | Haloperidol (n=203) | | Olanzapine (n=202) | | Quetiapine (n=202) | | Risperidone (n=202) | | Ziprasidone (n=201) | |
|---|---|---|---|---|---|---|---|---|---|---|---|---|
| | No. | % | No. | % | No. | % | No. | % | No. | % | No. | % |
| 1 (highly inappropriate) | 52 | 25.6 | 36 | 17.7 | 34 | 16.8 | 27 | 13.4 | 21 | 10.4 | 72 | 35.8 |
| 2 | 44 | 21.7 | 25 | 12.3 | 28 | 13.9 | 36 | 17.8 | 14 | 6.9 | 44 | 21.9 |
| 3 (uncertain) | 55 | 27.1 | 26 | 12.8 | 49 | 24.3 | 36 | 17.8 | 39 | 19.3 | 53 | 26.4 |
| 4 | 30 | 14.8 | 40 | 19.7 | 60 | 29.7 | 62 | 30.7 | 65 | 32.2 | 19 | 9.5 |
| 5 (highly appropriate) | 22 | 10.8 | 76 | 37.4 | 31 | 15.4 | 41 | 20.3 | 63 | 31.2 | 13 | 6.5 |
| Median | 3 | | 4 | | 3 | | 4 | | 4 | | 2 | |
| Mean | 2.6 | | 3.5 | | 3.1 | | 3.3 | | 3.7 | | 2.3 | |
| SD | 1.3 | | 1.5 | | 1.3 | | 1.3 | | 1.3 | | 1.2 | |

**1b.** The agitation is a NEW SYMPTOM. Assessment DOES NOT FIND a short-term reversible cause.

| Appropriateness of use | Aripiprazole (n=198) | | Haloperidol (n=199) | | Olanzapine (n=201) | | Quetiapine (n=200) | | Risperidone (n=199) | | Ziprasidone (n=198) | |
|---|---|---|---|---|---|---|---|---|---|---|---|---|
| | No. | % | No. | % | No. | % | No. | % | No. | % | No. | % |
| 1 (highly inappropriate) | 31 | 15.7 | 39 | 19.6 | 18 | 9.0 | 14 | 7.0 | 7 | 3.5 | 53 | 26.8 |
| 2 | 31 | 15.7 | 34 | 17.1 | 26 | 12.9 | 18 | 9.0 | 14 | 7.0 | 35 | 17.7 |
| 3 (uncertain) | 71 | 35.9 | 42 | 21.1 | 44 | 21.9 | 46 | 23.0 | 35 | 17.6 | 74 | 37.4 |
| 4 | 44 | 22.2 | 41 | 20.6 | 81 | 40.3 | 69 | 34.5 | 79 | 39.7 | 26 | 13.1 |
| 5 (highly appropriate) | 21 | 10.6 | 43 | 21.6 | 32 | 15.9 | 53 | 26.5 | 64 | 32.2 | 10 | 5.1 |
| Median | 3 | | 3 | | 4 | | 4 | | 4 | | 3 | |
| Mean | 3.0 | | 3.1 | | 3.4 | | 3.6 | | 3.9 | | 2.5 | |
| SD | 1.2 | | 1.4 | | 1.2 | | 1.2 | | 1 | | 1.2 | |

**1c.** The agitation is PERSISTENT or consists of repeated episodes. Assessment DOES NOT FIND a short-term reversible cause.

| Appropriateness of use | Aripiprazole (n=200) | | Haloperidol (n=201) | | Olanzapine (n=200) | | Quetiapine (n=201) | | Risperidone (n=199) | | Ziprasidone (n=198) | |
|---|---|---|---|---|---|---|---|---|---|---|---|---|
| | No. | % | No. | % | No. | % | No. | % | No. | % | No. | % |
| 1 (highly inappropriate) | 34 | 17.0 | 60 | 29.9 | 20 | 10.0 | 12 | 6.0 | 13 | 6.5 | 57 | 28.8 |
| 2 | 30 | 15.0 | 32 | 15.9 | 20 | 10.0 | 20 | 10.0 | 12 | 6.0 | 37 | 18.7 |
| 3 (uncertain) | 54 | 27.0 | 39 | 19.4 | 43 | 21.5 | 39 | 19.4 | 36 | 18.1 | 61 | 30.8 |
| 4 | 58 | 29.0 | 40 | 19.9 | 79 | 39.5 | 70 | 34.8 | 74 | 37.2 | 32 | 16.2 |
| 5 (highly appropriate) | 24 | 12.0 | 30 | 14.9 | 38 | 19.0 | 60 | 29.9 | 64 | 32.2 | 11 | 5.6 |
| Median | 3 | | 3 | | 4 | | 4 | | 4 | | 3 | |
| Mean | 3.1 | | 2.7 | | 3.5 | | 3.7 | | 3.8 | | 2.5 | |
| SD | 1.3 | | 1.4 | | 1.2 | | 1.2 | | 1.1 | | 1.2 | |

## 1a. Agitation is a new symptom from a short-term reversible cause

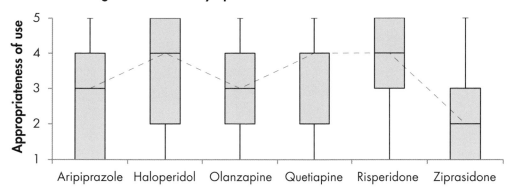

## 1b. Agitation is a new symptom without a short-term reversible cause

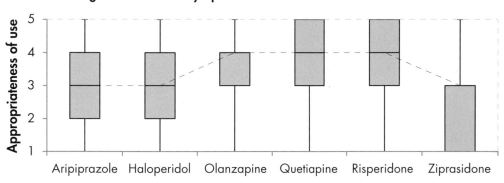

## 1c. Agitation is persistent or consists of repeated episodes

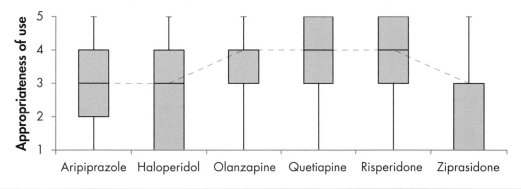

**FIGURE B–1.** Appropriateness of antipsychotics for the given clinical circumstance (1=highly inappropriate, 3=uncertain, 5=highly appropriate).

2. **Are there other antipsychotics (either first- or second-generation) that you think are highly appropriate (i.e., 5 on the 1–5 scale) for the clinical circumstances described in Question 1?**

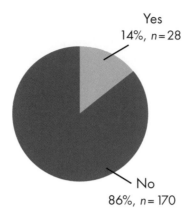

**FIGURE B–2.** Number of experts who thought that there are other antipsychotics (either first- or second-generation) that are highly appropriate (i.e., 5 on the 1-5 scale) for the clinical circumstances described in Question 1.

**3. Please specify the other antipsychotic(s) that you think are highly appropriate (i.e., 5 on the 1–5 scale) and check the appropriate clinical circumstance(s). Check all circumstances that apply.**

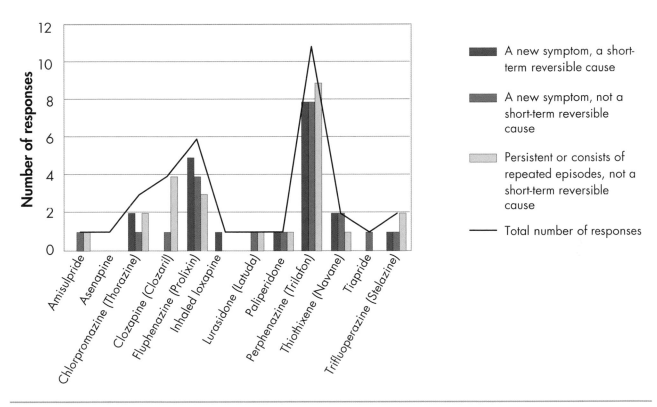

**FIGURE B–3.** Other antipsychotic(s) that the experts thought are highly appropriate (i.e., 5 on the 1–5 scale) for the given clinical circumstance(s) — checked all circumstances that apply.

## 4. NONDANGEROUS AGITATION—Please rate the appropriateness of each treatment for the given clinical circumstance.

**TABLE B–2.** Appropriateness of antipsychotics for the given clinical circumstance (rated using a 1–5 scale, where 1=highly inappropriate, 3=uncertain, and 5=highly appropriate)

**4a.** The agitation is a NEW SYMPTOM. Assessment SUGGESTS a short-term reversible cause of the agitation, such as acute delirium, medication side effects, or environmental causes.

| | Aripiprazole (n=198) | | Haloperidol (n=199) | | Olanzapine (n=198) | | Quetiapine (n=199) | | Risperidone (n=199) | | Ziprasidone (n=196) | |
|---|---|---|---|---|---|---|---|---|---|---|---|---|
| Appropriateness of use | No. | % | No. | % | No. | % | No. | % | No. | % | No. | % |
| 1 (highly inappropriate) | 97 | 49.0 | 78 | 39.2 | 76 | 38.4 | 64 | 32.2 | 58 | 29.2 | 115 | 58.7 |
| 2 | 38 | 19.2 | 41 | 20.6 | 37 | 18.7 | 36 | 18.1 | 38 | 19.1 | 32 | 16.3 |
| 3 (uncertain) | 37 | 18.7 | 30 | 15.1 | 34 | 17.2 | 42 | 21.1 | 38 | 19.1 | 27 | 13.8 |
| 4 | 18 | 9.1 | 29 | 14.6 | 39 | 19.7 | 32 | 16.1 | 44 | 22.1 | 15 | 7.7 |
| 5 (highly appropriate) | 8 | 4.0 | 21 | 10.6 | 12 | 6.1 | 25 | 12.6 | 21 | 10.6 | 7 | 3.6 |
| Median | 2 | | 2 | | 2 | | 2 | | 3 | | 1 | |
| Mean | 2.0 | | 2.4 | | 2.4 | | 2.6 | | 2.7 | | 1.8 | |
| SD | 1.2 | | 1.4 | | 1.3 | | 1.4 | | 1.4 | | 1.1 | |

**4b.** The agitation is a NEW SYMPTOM. Assessment DOES NOT FIND a short-term reversible cause.

| | Aripiprazole (n=193) | | Haloperidol (n=191) | | Olanzapine (n=192) | | Quetiapine (n=191) | | Risperidone (n=193) | | Ziprasidone (n=189) | |
|---|---|---|---|---|---|---|---|---|---|---|---|---|
| Appropriateness of use | No. | % | No. | % | No. | % | No. | % | No. | % | No. | % |
| 1 (highly inappropriate) | 71 | 36.8 | 74 | 38.7 | 59 | 30.7 | 48 | 25.1 | 45 | 23.3 | 96 | 50.8 |
| 2 | 39 | 20.2 | 48 | 25.1 | 41 | 21.4 | 37 | 19.4 | 37 | 19.2 | 35 | 18.5 |
| 3 (uncertain) | 53 | 27.5 | 33 | 17.3 | 41 | 21.4 | 44 | 23.0 | 46 | 23.8 | 38 | 20.1 |
| 4 | 25 | 13.0 | 23 | 12.0 | 43 | 22.4 | 39 | 20.4 | 51 | 26.4 | 16 | 8.5 |
| 5 (highly appropriate) | 5 | 2.6 | 13 | 6.8 | 8 | 4.2 | 23 | 12.0 | 14 | 7.3 | 4 | 2.1 |
| Median | 2 | | 2 | | 2 | | 3 | | 3 | | 1 | |
| Mean | 2.2 | | 2.2 | | 2.5 | | 2.7 | | 2.8 | | 1.9 | |
| SD | 1.2 | | 1.3 | | 1.2 | | 1.3 | | 1.3 | | 1.1 | |

**4c.** The agitation is PERSISTENT or consists of repeated episodes. Assessment DOES NOT FIND a short-term reversible cause.

| | Aripiprazole (n=193) | | Haloperidol (n=191) | | Olanzapine (n=191) | | Quetiapine (n=191) | | Risperidone (n=192) | | Ziprasidone (n=189) | |
|---|---|---|---|---|---|---|---|---|---|---|---|---|
| Appropriateness of use | No. | % | No. | % | No. | % | No. | % | No. | % | No. | % |
| 1 (highly inappropriate) | 62 | 32.1 | 81 | 42.4 | 59 | 30.9 | 37 | 19.4 | 43 | 22.4 | 88 | 46.6 |
| 2 | 33 | 17.1 | 39 | 20.4 | 31 | 16.2 | 36 | 18.9 | 32 | 16.7 | 28 | 14.8 |
| 3 (uncertain) | 63 | 32.6 | 35 | 18.3 | 42 | 22.0 | 47 | 24.6 | 42 | 21.9 | 49 | 25.9 |
| 4 | 30 | 15.5 | 27 | 14.1 | 46 | 24.1 | 44 | 23.0 | 56 | 29.2 | 20 | 10.6 |
| 5 (highly appropriate) | 5 | 2.6 | 9 | 4.7 | 13 | 6.8 | 27 | 14.1 | 19 | 9.9 | 4 | 2.1 |
| Median | 3 | | 2 | | 3 | | 3 | | 3 | | 2 | |
| Mean | 2.4 | | 2.2 | | 2.6 | | 2.9 | | 2.9 | | 2.1 | |
| SD | 1.2 | | 1.3 | | 1.3 | | 1.3 | | 1.3 | | 1.2 | |

## 4a. Agitation is a new symptom from a short-term reversible cause

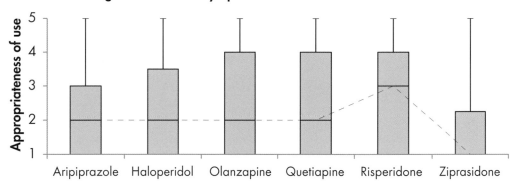

## 4b. Agitation is a new symptom without a short-term reversible cause

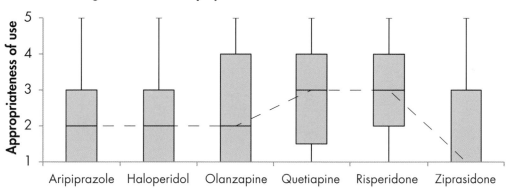

## 4c. Agitation is persistent or consists of repeated episodes

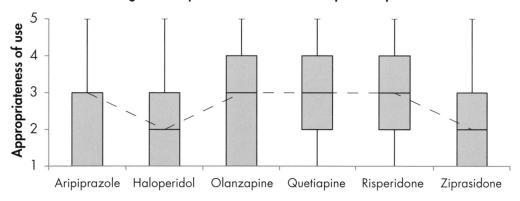

**FIGURE B–4.** Appropriateness of antipsychotics for the given clinical circumstance (1 = highly inappropriate, 3 = uncertain, 5 = highly appropriate).

5. **Are there other antipsychotics (either first- or second-generation) that you think are highly appropriate (i.e., 5 on the 1–5 scale) for the clinical circumstances described in Question 4?**

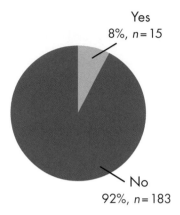

**FIGURE B–5.**   Number of experts who thought that there are other antipsychotics (either first- or second-generation) that are highly appropriate (i.e., 5 on the 1–5 scale) for the clinical circumstances described in Question 4.

6. **Please specify the other antipsychotic(s) that you think are highly appropriate (i.e., 5 on the 1–5 scale) and check the appropriate clinical circumstance(s). Check all circumstances that apply.**

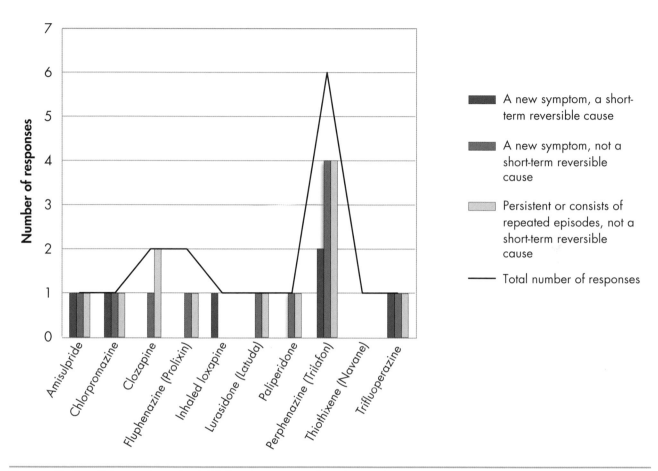

**FIGURE B–6.** Other antipsychotic(s) that the experts thought are highly appropriate (i.e., 5 on the 1–5 scale) for the given clinical circumstance(s)—checked all circumstances that apply.

## 7. DANGEROUS PSYCHOSIS—Please rate the appropriateness of each treatment for the given clinical circumstance.

**TABLE B–3.** Appropriateness of antipsychotics for the given clinical circumstance (rated using a 1–5 scale, where 1 = highly inappropriate, 3 = uncertain, and 5 = highly appropriate)

**7a.** The psychosis is a NEW SYMPTOM. Assessment SUGGESTS a short-term reversible cause of the agitation, such as acute delirium, medication side effects, or environmental causes.

| | Aripiprazole (n=185) | | Haloperidol (n=187) | | Olanzapine (n=185) | | Quetiapine (n=186) | | Risperidone (n=187) | | Ziprasidone (n=182) | |
|---|---|---|---|---|---|---|---|---|---|---|---|---|
| Appropriateness of use | No. | % | No. | % | No. | % | No. | % | No. | % | No. | % |
| 1 (highly inappropriate) | 43 | 23.2 | 24 | 12.8 | 20 | 10.8 | 19 | 10.2 | 10 | 5.4 | 55 | 30.2 |
| 2 | 25 | 13.5 | 15 | 8.0 | 14 | 7.6 | 19 | 10.2 | 9 | 4.8 | 32 | 17.6 |
| 3 (uncertain) | 38 | 20.5 | 27 | 14.4 | 34 | 18.4 | 36 | 19.4 | 27 | 14.4 | 51 | 28.0 |
| 4 | 38 | 20.5 | 36 | 19.3 | 61 | 33.0 | 54 | 29.0 | 48 | 25.7 | 22 | 12.1 |
| 5 (highly appropriate) | 41 | 22.2 | 85 | 45.5 | 56 | 30.3 | 58 | 31.2 | 93 | 49.7 | 22 | 12.1 |
| Median | 3 | | 4 | | 4 | | 4 | | 4 | | 3 | |
| Mean | 3.0 | | 3.8 | | 3.6 | | 3.6 | | 4.1 | | 2.6 | |
| SD | 1.5 | | 1.4 | | 1.3 | | 1.3 | | 1.1 | | 1.3 | |

**7b.** The psychosis is a NEW SYMPTOM. Assessment DOES NOT FIND a short-term reversible cause.

| | Aripiprazole (n=181) | | Haloperidol (n=186) | | Olanzapine (n=185) | | Quetiapine (n=183) | | Risperidone (n=181) | | Ziprasidone (n=183) | |
|---|---|---|---|---|---|---|---|---|---|---|---|---|
| Appropriateness of use | No. | % | No. | % | No. | % | No. | % | No. | % | No. | % |
| 1 (highly inappropriate) | 30 | 16.6 | 34 | 18.3 | 18 | 9.7 | 11 | 6.0 | 6 | 3.3 | 52 | 28.4 |
| 2 | 25 | 13.8 | 17 | 9.1 | 8 | 4.3 | 13 | 7.1 | 7 | 3.9 | 24 | 13.1 |
| 3 (uncertain) | 37 | 20.4 | 32 | 17.2 | 33 | 17.8 | 31 | 16.9 | 22 | 12.2 | 57 | 31.2 |
| 4 | 41 | 22.7 | 38 | 20.4 | 59 | 31.9 | 57 | 31.2 | 53 | 29.3 | 27 | 14.8 |
| 5 (highly appropriate) | 48 | 26.5 | 65 | 35.0 | 67 | 36.2 | 71 | 38.8 | 93 | 51.4 | 23 | 12.6 |
| Median | 3 | | 4 | | 4 | | 4 | | 5 | | 3 | |
| Mean | 3.3 | | 3.4 | | 3.8 | | 3.9 | | 4.2 | | 2.7 | |
| SD | 1.4 | | 1.5 | | 1.2 | | 1.2 | | 1 | | 1.4 | |

**7c.** The psychosis is PERSISTENT or consists of repeated episodes. Assessment DOES NOT FIND a short-term reversible cause.

| | Aripiprazole (n=182) | | Haloperidol (n=187) | | Olanzapine (n=184) | | Quetiapine (n=182) | | Risperidone (n=183) | | Ziprasidone (n=182) | |
|---|---|---|---|---|---|---|---|---|---|---|---|---|
| Appropriateness of use | No. | (%) | No. | (%) | No. | (%) | No. | (%) | No. | (%) | No. | (%) |
| 1 (highly inappropriate) | 27 | 14.8 | 44 | 23.5 | 18 | 9.8 | 12 | 6.6 | 9 | 4.9 | 50 | 27.5 |
| 2 | 17 | 9.3 | 24 | 12.8 | 14 | 7.6 | 5 | 2.8 | 6 | 3.3 | 21 | 11.5 |
| 3 (uncertain) | 39 | 21.4 | 35 | 18.7 | 22 | 12.0 | 35 | 19.2 | 18 | 9.8 | 56 | 30.8 |
| 4 | 45 | 24.7 | 33 | 17.7 | 59 | 32.1 | 48 | 26.4 | 56 | 30.6 | 29 | 15.9 |
| 5 (highly appropriate) | 54 | 29.7 | 51 | 27.3 | 71 | 38.6 | 82 | 45.1 | 94 | 51.4 | 26 | 14.3 |
| Median | 4 | | 3 | | 4 | | 4 | | 5 | | 3 | |
| Mean | 3.5 | | 3.1 | | 3.8 | | 4.0 | | 4.2 | | 2.8 | |
| SD | 1.4 | | 1.5 | | 1.3 | | 1.2 | | 1.1 | | 1.4 | |

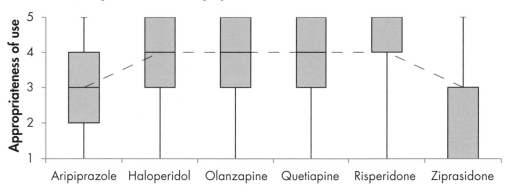

**7a. Psychosis is a new symptom from a short-term reversible cause**

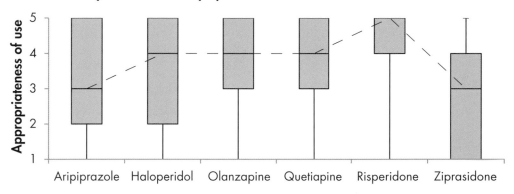

**7b. Psychosis is a new symptom without a short-term reversible cause**

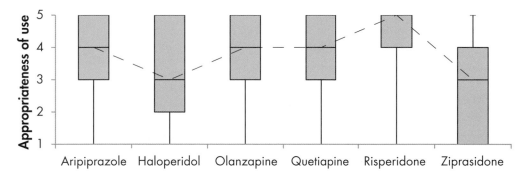

**7c. Psychosis is persistent or consists of repeated episodes**

**FIGURE B–7.** Appropriateness of antipsychotics for the given clinical circumstance (1 = highly inappropriate, 3 = uncertain, 5 = highly appropriate).

8. **Are there other antipsychotics (either first- or second-generation) that you think are highly appropriate (i.e., 5 on the 1–5 scale) for the clinical circumstances described in Question 7?**

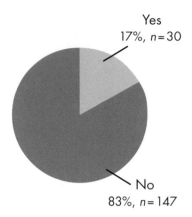

**FIGURE B–8.** Number of experts who thought that there are other antipsychotics (either first- or second-generation) that are highly appropriate (i.e., 5 on the 1–5 scale) for the clinical circumstances described in Question 7.

**9. Please specify the other antipsychotic(s) that you think are highly appropriate (i.e., 5 on the 1–5 scale) and check the appropriate clinical circumstance(s). Check all circumstances that apply.**

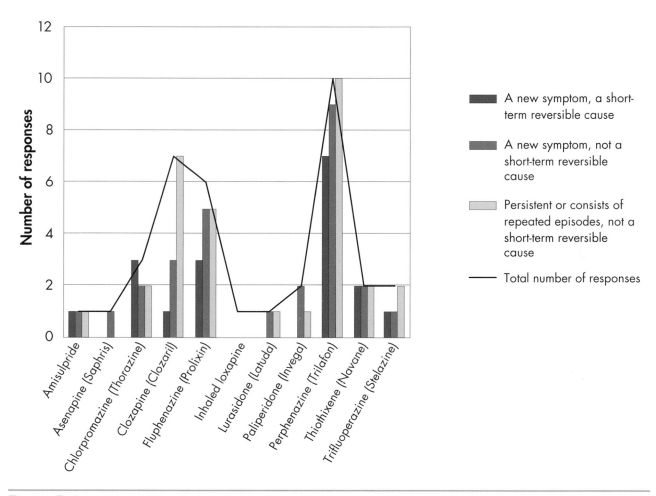

**FIGURE B–9.** Other antipsychotic(s) that the experts thought are highly appropriate (i.e., 5 on the 1-5 scale) for the given clinical circumstance(s)—checked all circumstances that apply.

## 10. NONDANGEROUS PSYCHOSIS—Please rate the appropriateness of each treatment for the given clinical circumstance.

**TABLE B–4.** Appropriateness of antipsychotics for the given clinical circumstance (rated using a 1–5 scale where 1 = highly inappropriate, 3 = uncertain, and 5 = highly appropriate)

**10a. The psychosis is a NEW SYMPTOM. Assessment SUGGESTS a short-term reversible cause of the agitation, such as acute delirium, medication side effects, or environmental causes.**

| Appropriateness of use | Aripiprazole (n=187) | | Haloperidol (n=188) | | Olanzapine (n=187) | | Quetiapine (n=187) | | Risperidone (n=186) | | Ziprasidone (n=181) | |
|---|---|---|---|---|---|---|---|---|---|---|---|---|
| | No. | % | No. | % | No. | % | No. | % | No. | % | No. | % |
| 1 (highly inappropriate) | 78 | 41.7 | 67 | 35.6 | 57 | 30.5 | 50 | 26.7 | 43 | 23.1 | 91 | 50.3 |
| 2 | 25 | 13.4 | 36 | 19.2 | 34 | 18.2 | 37 | 19.8 | 33 | 17.7 | 30 | 16.6 |
| 3 (uncertain) | 48 | 25.7 | 27 | 14.4 | 38 | 20.3 | 38 | 20.3 | 34 | 18.3 | 39 | 21.6 |
| 4 | 22 | 11.8 | 35 | 18.6 | 39 | 20.9 | 39 | 20.9 | 45 | 24.2 | 11 | 6.1 |
| 5 (highly appropriate) | 14 | 7.5 | 23 | 12.2 | 19 | 10.2 | 23 | 12.3 | 31 | 16.7 | 10 | 5.5 |
| Median | 2 | | 2 | | 3 | | 3 | | 3 | | 1 | |
| Mean | 2.3 | | 2.5 | | 2.6 | | 2.7 | | 2.9 | | 2.0 | |
| SD | 1.3 | | 1.4 | | 1.4 | | 1.4 | | 1.4 | | 1.2 | |

**10b. The psychosis is a NEW SYMPTOM. Assessment DOES NOT FIND a short-term reversible cause.**

| Appropriateness of use | Aripiprazole (n=184) | | Haloperidol (n=183) | | Olanzapine (n=183) | | Quetiapine (n=184) | | Risperidone (n=181) | | Ziprasidone (n=182) | |
|---|---|---|---|---|---|---|---|---|---|---|---|---|
| | No. | % | No. | % | No. | % | No. | % | No. | % | No. | % |
| 1 (highly inappropriate) | 59 | 32.1 | 67 | 36.6 | 43 | 23.5 | 37 | 20.1 | 36 | 19.9 | 74 | 40.7 |
| 2 | 23 | 12.5 | 34 | 18.6 | 32 | 17.5 | 33 | 17.9 | 27 | 14.9 | 31 | 17.0 |
| 3 (uncertain) | 49 | 26.6 | 33 | 18.0 | 35 | 19.1 | 45 | 24.5 | 43 | 23.8 | 44 | 24.2 |
| 4 | 36 | 19.6 | 29 | 15.9 | 51 | 27.9 | 42 | 22.8 | 45 | 24.9 | 20 | 11.0 |
| 5 (highly appropriate) | 17 | 9.2 | 20 | 10.9 | 22 | 12.0 | 27 | 14.7 | 30 | 16.6 | 13 | 7.1 |
| Median | 3 | | 2 | | 3 | | 3 | | 3 | | 2 | |
| Mean | 2.6 | | 2.5 | | 2.9 | | 2.9 | | 3.0 | | 2.3 | |
| SD | 1.4 | | 1.4 | | 1.4 | | 1.3 | | 1.4 | | 1.3 | |

**10c. The psychosis is PERSISTENT or consists of repeated episodes. Assessment DOES NOT FIND a short-term reversible cause.**

| Appropriateness of use | Aripiprazole (n=182) | | Haloperidol (n=183) | | Olanzapine (n=184) | | Quetiapine (n=184) | | Risperidone (n=182) | | Ziprasidone (n=179) | |
|---|---|---|---|---|---|---|---|---|---|---|---|---|
| | No. | % | No. | % | No. | % | No. | % | No. | % | No. | % |
| 1 (highly inappropriate) | 49 | 26.9 | 67 | 36.6 | 39 | 21.2 | 32 | 17.4 | 33 | 18.1 | 70 | 39.1 |
| 2 | 29 | 15.9 | 44 | 24.0 | 37 | 20.1 | 37 | 20.1 | 27 | 14.8 | 38 | 21.2 |
| 3 (uncertain) | 42 | 23.1 | 28 | 15.3 | 31 | 16.9 | 38 | 20.7 | 38 | 20.9 | 42 | 23.5 |
| 4 | 44 | 24.2 | 23 | 12.6 | 53 | 28.8 | 44 | 23.9 | 50 | 27.5 | 15 | 8.4 |
| 5 (highly appropriate) | 18 | 9.9 | 21 | 11.5 | 24 | 13.0 | 33 | 17.9 | 34 | 18.7 | 14 | 7.8 |
| Median | 3 | | 2 | | 3 | | 3 | | 3 | | 2 | |
| Mean | 2.7 | | 2.4 | | 2.9 | | 3.0 | | 3.1 | | 2.2 | |
| SD | 1.3 | | 1.4 | | 1.4 | | 1.4 | | 1.4 | | 1.3 | |

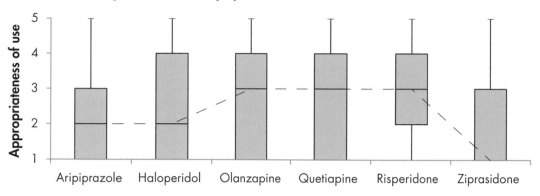

**10a. Psychosis is a new symptom from a short-term reversible cause**

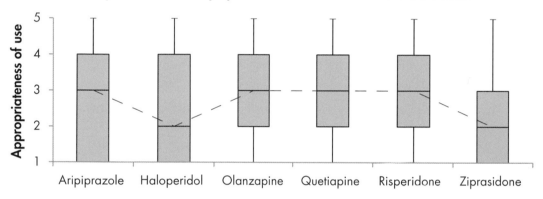

**10b. Psychosis is a new symptom without a short-term reversible cause**

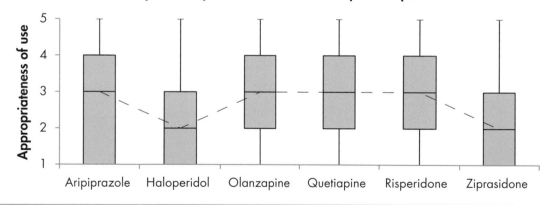

**10c. Psychosis is persistent or consists of repeated episodes**

**FIGURE B–10.** Appropriateness of antipsychotics for the given clinical circumstance (1 = highly inappropriate, 3 = uncertain, 5 = highly appropriate).

**11. Are there other antipsychotics (either first- or second-generation) that you think are highly appropriate (i.e., 5 on the 1–5 scale) for the clinical circumstances described in Question 10?**

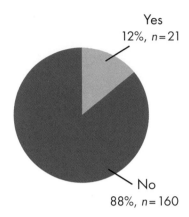

Yes
12%, *n* = 21

No
88%, *n* = 160

**FIGURE B–11.**  Number of experts who thought that there are other antipsychotics (either first- or second-generation) that are highly appropriate (i.e., 5 on the 1–5 scale) for the clinical circumstances described in Question 10.

**12. Please specify the other antipsychotic(s) that you think are highly appropriate (i.e., 5 on the 1–5 scale) and check the appropriate clinical circumstance(s). Check all circumstances that apply.**

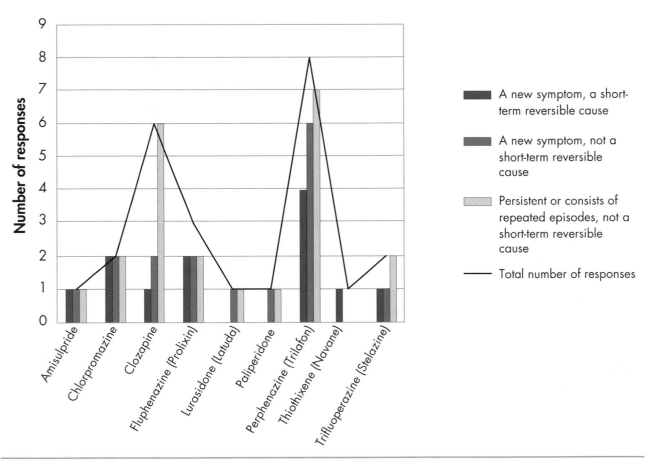

**FIGURE B–12.** Other antipsychotic(s) that the experts thought are highly appropriate (i.e., 5 on the 1–5 scale) for the given clinical circumstance(s)—checked all circumstances that apply.

# Section II: Duration of Treatment

## 13. If a patient with dementia has been stabilized on an antipsychotic medication for the treatment of DANGEROUS AGITATION, what duration of treatment is usually optimal?

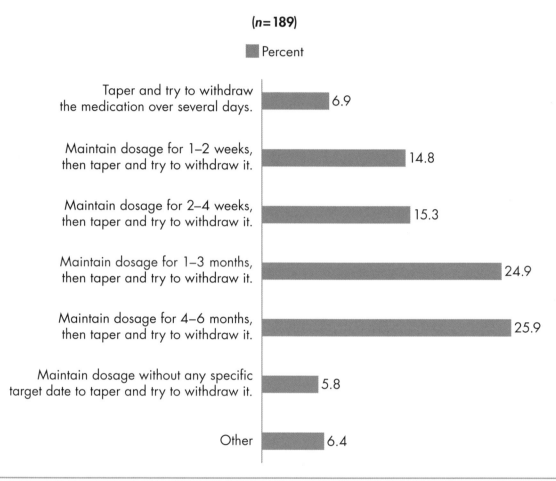

(*n*=189)

■ Percent

| | |
|---|---|
| Taper and try to withdraw the medication over several days. | 6.9 |
| Maintain dosage for 1–2 weeks, then taper and try to withdraw it. | 14.8 |
| Maintain dosage for 2–4 weeks, then taper and try to withdraw it. | 15.3 |
| Maintain dosage for 1–3 months, then taper and try to withdraw it. | 24.9 |
| Maintain dosage for 4–6 months, then taper and try to withdraw it. | 25.9 |
| Maintain dosage without any specific target date to taper and try to withdraw it. | 5.8 |
| Other | 6.4 |

**FIGURE B–13.** Optimal duration if a patient with dementia has been stabilized on an antipsychotic medication for the treatment of dangerous agitation.

APA Practice Guidelines

## 14. If a patient with dementia has been stabilized on an antipsychotic medication for the treatment of NONDANGEROUS AGITATION, what duration of treatment is usually optimal?

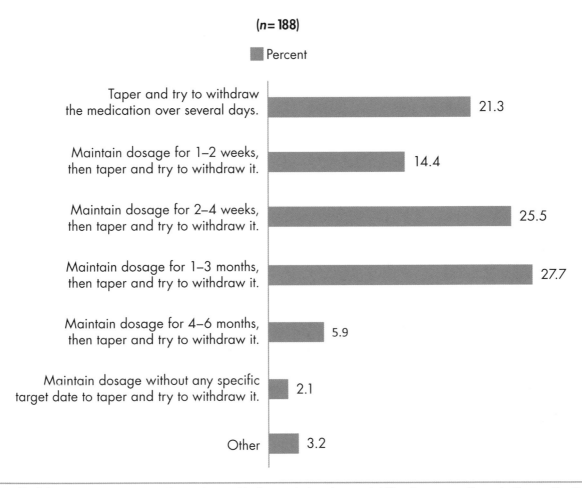

(*n* = 188)

■ Percent

| | |
|---|---|
| Taper and try to withdraw the medication over several days. | 21.3 |
| Maintain dosage for 1–2 weeks, then taper and try to withdraw it. | 14.4 |
| Maintain dosage for 2–4 weeks, then taper and try to withdraw it. | 25.5 |
| Maintain dosage for 1–3 months, then taper and try to withdraw it. | 27.7 |
| Maintain dosage for 4–6 months, then taper and try to withdraw it. | 5.9 |
| Maintain dosage without any specific target date to taper and try to withdraw it. | 2.1 |
| Other | 3.2 |

**FIGURE B–14.**    Optimal duration if a patient with dementia has been stabilized on an antipsychotic medication for the treatment of nondangerous agitation.

## 15. If a patient with dementia has been stabilized on an antipsychotic medication for the treatment of DANGEROUS PSYCHOSIS, what duration of treatment is usually optimal?

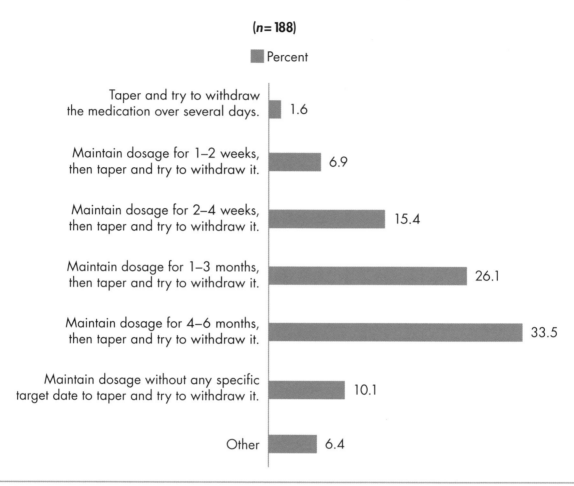

**FIGURE B–15.** Optimal duration if a patient with dementia has been stabilized on an antipsychotic medication for the treatment of dangerous psychosis.

## 16. If a patient with dementia has been stabilized on an antipsychotic medication for the treatment of NONDANGEROUS PSYCHOSIS, what duration of treatment is optimal?

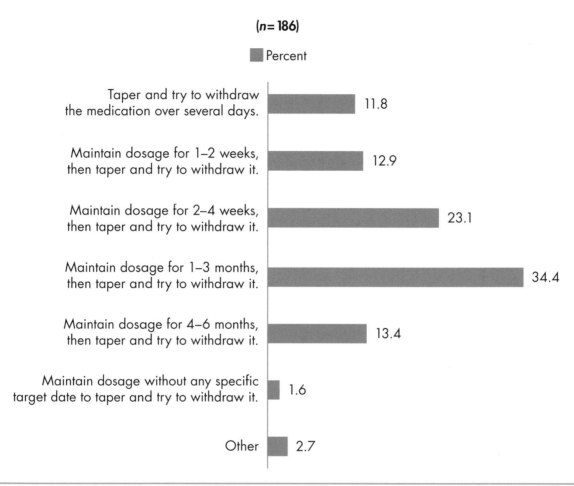

FIGURE B–16. Optimal duration if a patient with dementia has been stabilized on an antipsychotic medication for the treatment of nondangerous psychosis.

**Optimal duration of treatment**

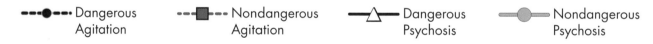

FIGURE B–17. Comparision of optimal duration of an antipsychotic medication for the treatment of dangerous and nondangerous agitation, and dangerous and nondangerous psychosis, if a patient with dementia has been stabilized on the medication.

# Section III: Clinical Experience Using Antipsychotics in Patients With Dementia

**17. Please check any of the following disciplines that describe your own professional training, background, and focus of practice or research:**

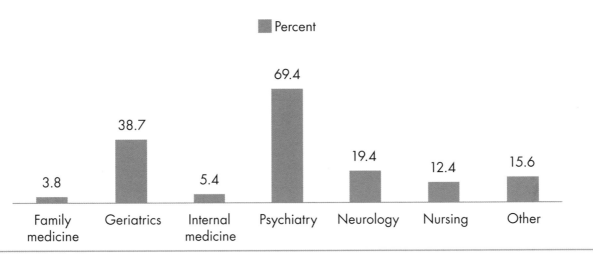

**FIGURE B–18.** Disciplines that describe experts' professional training, background, and focus of practice or research—checked any that applied.

**18. Not including training, how many years have you been in practice?**

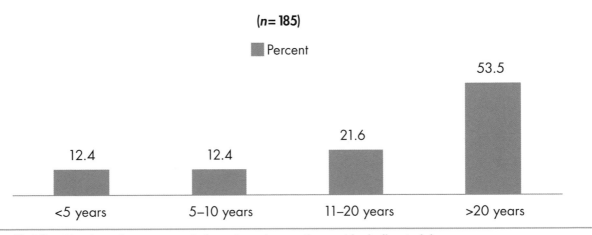

**FIGURE B–19.** Number of years experts have been in practice, not including training.

## 19. Please indicate your degree of expertise in the treatment of patients with dementia, including pharmacological treatment of behavioral symptoms.

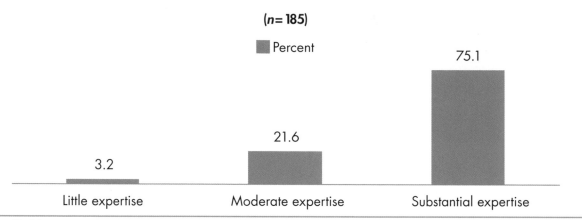

**FIGURE B–20.** Experts' degree of expertise in the treatment of patients with dementia, including pharmacological treatment of behavioral symptoms.

## 20. Do you currently treat patients with dementia?

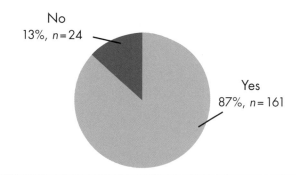

**FIGURE B–21.** Number of experts who currently treat patients with dementia.

## 21. To what extent have the following potential adverse effects of antipsychotics decreased your use of them to treat agitation or psychosis in your patients with dementia WITHIN THE PAST YEAR?

TABLE B–5. The extent of decreased use of antipsychotics due to the potential adverse effects in the treatment of agitation or psychosis in patients with dementia within the past year (1 = not at all, 3 = somewhat, 5 = very much)

### 21a. AKATHISIA

| Extent of decreased use | Aripiprazole (n=146) | | Haloperidol (n=147) | | Olanzapine (n=142) | | Quetiapine (n=145) | | Risperidone (n=145) | | Ziprasidone (n=142) | |
|---|---|---|---|---|---|---|---|---|---|---|---|---|
| | No. | % | No. | % | No. | % | No. | % | No. | % | No. | % |
| 1 (not at all) | 46 | 31.5 | 31 | 21.1 | 50 | 35.2 | 77 | 53.1 | 38 | 26.2 | 56 | 39.4 |
| 2 | 21 | 14.4 | 16 | 10.9 | 38 | 26.8 | 34 | 23.5 | 29 | 20.0 | 24 | 16.9 |
| 3 (somewhat) | 33 | 22.6 | 33 | 22.5 | 37 | 26.1 | 22 | 15.2 | 38 | 26.2 | 43 | 30.3 |
| 4 | 34 | 23.3 | 39 | 26.5 | 11 | 7.8 | 10 | 6.9 | 30 | 20.7 | 12 | 8.5 |
| 5 (very much) | 12 | 8.2 | 28 | 19.1 | 6 | 4.2 | 2 | 1.4 | 10 | 6.9 | 7 | 4.9 |
| Median | 3 | | 3 | | 2 | | 1 | | 3 | | 2 | |
| Mean | 2.6 | | 3.1 | | 2.2 | | 1.8 | | 2.6 | | 2.2 | |
| SD | 1.4 | | 1.4 | | 1.1 | | 1.0 | | 1.3 | | 1.2 | |

### 21b. ANTICHOLINERGIC EFFECTS

| Extent of decreased use | Aripiprazole (n=145) | | Haloperidol (n=146) | | Olanzapine (n=143) | | Quetiapine (n=147) | | Risperidone (n=145) | | Ziprasidone (n=143) | |
|---|---|---|---|---|---|---|---|---|---|---|---|---|
| | No. | % | No. | % | No. | % | No. | % | No. | % | No. | % |
| 1 (not at all) | 94 | 64.8 | 72 | 49.3 | 41 | 28.7 | 60 | 40.8 | 66 | 45.5 | 82 | 57.3 |
| 2 | 24 | 16.6 | 24 | 16.4 | 31 | 21.7 | 33 | 22.5 | 37 | 25.5 | 22 | 15.4 |
| 3 (somewhat) | 16 | 11.0 | 24 | 16.4 | 39 | 27.3 | 31 | 21.1 | 23 | 15.9 | 29 | 20.3 |
| 4 | 9 | 6.2 | 14 | 9.6 | 24 | 16.8 | 16 | 10.9 | 13 | 9.0 | 8 | 5.6 |
| 5 (very much) | 2 | 1.4 | 12 | 8.2 | 8 | 5.6 | 7 | 4.8 | 6 | 4.1 | 2 | 1.4 |
| Median | 1 | | 2 | | 2 | | 2 | | 2 | | 1 | |
| Mean | 1.6 | | 2.1 | | 2.5 | | 2.2 | | 2.0 | | 1.8 | |
| SD | 1.0 | | 1.3 | | 1.2 | | 1.2 | | 1.2 | | 1.0 | |

### 21c. CARDIAC EFFECTS

| Extent of decreased use | Aripiprazole (n=141) | | Haloperidol (n=144) | | Olanzapine (n=143) | | Quetiapine (n=143) | | Risperidone (n=142) | | Ziprasidone (n=143) | |
|---|---|---|---|---|---|---|---|---|---|---|---|---|
| | No. | % | No. | % | No. | % | No. | % | No. | % | No. | % |
| 1 (not at all) | 81 | 57.5 | 56 | 38.9 | 55 | 38.5 | 58 | 40.6 | 55 | 38.7 | 43 | 30.1 |
| 2 | 16 | 11.4 | 27 | 18.8 | 24 | 16.8 | 27 | 18.9 | 27 | 19.0 | 13 | 9.1 |
| 3 (somewhat) | 21 | 14.9 | 25 | 17.4 | 34 | 23.8 | 31 | 21.7 | 29 | 20.4 | 34 | 23.8 |
| 4 | 15 | 10.6 | 21 | 14.6 | 21 | 14.7 | 19 | 13.3 | 21 | 14.8 | 25 | 17.5 |
| 5 (very much) | 8 | 5.7 | 15 | 10.4 | 9 | 6.3 | 8 | 5.6 | 10 | 7.0 | 28 | 19.6 |
| Median | 1 | | 2 | | 2 | | 2 | | 2 | | 3 | |
| Mean | 2.0 | | 2.4 | | 2.3 | | 2.2 | | 2.3 | | 2.9 | |
| SD | 1.3 | | 1.4 | | 1.3 | | 1.3 | | 1.3 | | 1.5 | |

**TABLE B–5.** The extent of decreased use of antipsychotics due to the potential adverse effects in the treatment of agitation or psychosis in patients with dementia within the past year (1 = not at all, 3 = somewhat, 5 = very much) *(continued)*

### 21d. DEATH

| Extent of decreased use | Aripiprazole (n=148) No. | % | Haloperidol (n=149) No. | % | Olanzapine (n=148) No. | % | Quetiapine (n=148) No. | % | Risperidone (n=145) No. | % | Ziprasidone (n=145) No. | % |
|---|---|---|---|---|---|---|---|---|---|---|---|---|
| 1 (not at all) | 73 | 49.3 | 62 | 41.6 | 59 | 39.9 | 63 | 42.6 | 59 | 40.7 | 58 | 40.0 |
| 2 | 13 | 8.8 | 17 | 11.4 | 17 | 11.5 | 18 | 12.2 | 18 | 12.4 | 13 | 9.0 |
| 3 (somewhat) | 31 | 21.0 | 25 | 16.8 | 36 | 24.3 | 36 | 24.3 | 32 | 22.1 | 37 | 25.5 |
| 4 | 17 | 11.5 | 24 | 16.1 | 17 | 11.5 | 17 | 11.5 | 20 | 13.8 | 19 | 13.1 |
| 5 (very much) | 14 | 9.5 | 21 | 14.1 | 19 | 12.8 | 14 | 9.5 | 16 | 11.0 | 18 | 12.4 |
| Median | 2 | | 2 | | 2 | | 2 | | 2 | | 3 | |
| Mean | 2.2 | | 2.5 | | 2.5 | | 2.3 | | 2.4 | | 2.5 | |
| SD | 1.4 | | 1.5 | | 1.4 | | 1.4 | | 1.4 | | 1.4 | |

### 21e. DRUG-INDUCED PARKINSONISM

| Extent of decreased use | Aripiprazole (n=145) No. | % | Haloperidol (n=148) No. | % | Olanzapine (n=143) No. | % | Quetiapine (n=146) No. | % | Risperidone (n=147) No. | % | Ziprasidone (n=141) No. | % |
|---|---|---|---|---|---|---|---|---|---|---|---|---|
| 1 (not at all) | 65 | 44.8 | 20 | 13.5 | 46 | 32.2 | 79 | 54.1 | 23 | 15.7 | 61 | 43.3 |
| 2 | 23 | 15.9 | 12 | 8.1 | 30 | 21.0 | 35 | 24.0 | 18 | 12.2 | 30 | 21.3 |
| 3 (somewhat) | 35 | 24.1 | 33 | 22.3 | 44 | 30.8 | 23 | 15.8 | 53 | 36.1 | 32 | 22.7 |
| 4 | 15 | 10.3 | 34 | 23.0 | 16 | 11.2 | 6 | 4.1 | 34 | 23.1 | 11 | 7.8 |
| 5 (very much) | 7 | 4.8 | 49 | 33.1 | 7 | 4.9 | 3 | 2.1 | 19 | 12.9 | 7 | 5.0 |
| Median | 2 | | 4 | | 2 | | 1 | | 3 | | 2 | |
| Mean | 2.1 | | 3.5 | | 2.4 | | 1.8 | | 3.1 | | 2.1 | |
| SD | 1.2 | | 1.4 | | 1.2 | | 1.0 | | 1.2 | | 1.2 | |

### 21f. METABOLIC EFFECTS, EXCLUDING WEIGHT GAIN

| Extent of decreased use | Aripiprazole (n=143) No. | % | Haloperidol (n=145) No. | % | Olanzapine (n=149) No. | % | Quetiapine (n=147) No. | % | Risperidone (n=146) No. | % | Ziprasidone (n=143) No. | % |
|---|---|---|---|---|---|---|---|---|---|---|---|---|
| 1 (not at all) | 75 | 52.5 | 79 | 54.5 | 28 | 18.8 | 43 | 29.3 | 45 | 30.8 | 74 | 51.8 |
| 2 | 31 | 21.7 | 31 | 21.4 | 18 | 12.1 | 26 | 17.7 | 37 | 25.3 | 30 | 21.0 |
| 3 (somewhat) | 22 | 15.4 | 20 | 13.8 | 32 | 21.5 | 38 | 25.9 | 39 | 26.7 | 29 | 20.3 |
| 4 | 12 | 8.4 | 10 | 6.9 | 35 | 23.5 | 28 | 19.1 | 22 | 15.1 | 7 | 4.9 |
| 5 (very much) | 3 | 2.1 | 5 | 3.5 | 36 | 24.2 | 12 | 8.2 | 3 | 2.1 | 3 | 2.1 |
| Median | 1 | | 1 | | 3 | | 3 | | 2 | | 1 | |
| Mean | 1.9 | | 1.8 | | 3.2 | | 2.6 | | 2.3 | | 1.8 | |
| SD | 1.1 | | 1.1 | | 1.4 | | 1.3 | | 1.1 | | 1.0 | |

### 21g. NEUROLEPTIC MALIGNANT SYNDROME

| Extent of decreased use | Aripiprazole (n=148) | | Haloperidol (n=149) | | Olanzapine (n=144) | | Quetiapine (n=146) | | Risperidone (n=146) | | Ziprasidone (n=142) | |
|---|---|---|---|---|---|---|---|---|---|---|---|---|
| | No. | % | No. | % | No. | % | No. | % | No. | % | No. | % |
| 1 (not at all) | 93 | 62.8 | 72 | 48.3 | 86 | 59.7 | 95 | 65.1 | 82 | 56.2 | 87 | 61.3 |
| 2 | 20 | 13.5 | 19 | 12.8 | 20 | 13.9 | 20 | 13.7 | 24 | 16.4 | 22 | 15.5 |
| 3 (somewhat) | 18 | 12.2 | 22 | 14.8 | 24 | 16.7 | 23 | 15.8 | 21 | 14.4 | 24 | 16.9 |
| 4 | 14 | 9.5 | 25 | 16.8 | 9 | 6.3 | 7 | 4.8 | 15 | 10.3 | 7 | 4.9 |
| 5 (very much) | 3 | 2.0 | 11 | 7.4 | 5 | 3.5 | 1 | 0.7 | 4 | 2.7 | 2 | 1.4 |
| Median | 1 | | 2 | | 1 | | 1 | | 1 | | 1 | |
| Mean | 1.7 | | 2.2 | | 1.8 | | 1.6 | | 1.9 | | 1.7 | |
| SD | 1.1 | | 1.4 | | 1.1 | | 1.0 | | 1.2 | | 1.0 | |

### 21h. STROKE

| Extent of decreased use | Aripiprazole (n=148) | | Haloperidol (n=150) | | Olanzapine (n=148) | | Quetiapine (n=148) | | Risperidone (n=148) | | Ziprasidone (n=145) | |
|---|---|---|---|---|---|---|---|---|---|---|---|---|
| | No. | % | No. | % | No. | % | No. | % | No. | % | No. | % |
| 1 (not at all) | 71 | 48.0 | 62 | 41.3 | 55 | 37.2 | 61 | 41.2 | 55 | 37.2 | 62 | 42.8 |
| 2 | 22 | 14.9 | 21 | 14.0 | 21 | 14.2 | 26 | 17.6 | 29 | 19.6 | 23 | 15.9 |
| 3 (somewhat) | 30 | 20.3 | 32 | 21.3 | 36 | 24.3 | 34 | 23.0 | 33 | 22.3 | 33 | 22.8 |
| 4 | 17 | 11.5 | 21 | 14.0 | 26 | 17.6 | 21 | 14.2 | 23 | 15.5 | 18 | 12.4 |
| 5 (very much) | 8 | 5.4 | 14 | 9.3 | 10 | 6.8 | 6 | 4.1 | 8 | 5.4 | 9 | 6.2 |
| Median | 2 | | 2 | | 2 | | 2 | | 2 | | 2 | |
| Mean | 2.1 | | 2.4 | | 2.4 | | 2.2 | | 2.3 | | 2.2 | |
| SD | 1.3 | | 1.4 | | 1.3 | | 1.2 | | 1.3 | | 1.3 | |

### 21i. WEIGHT GAIN

| Extent of decreased use | Aripiprazole (n=145) | | Haloperidol (n=147) | | Olanzapine (n=147) | | Quetiapine (n=149) | | Risperidone (n=146) | | Ziprasidone (n=143) | |
|---|---|---|---|---|---|---|---|---|---|---|---|---|
| | No. | % | No. | % | No. | % | No. | % | No. | % | No. | % |
| 1 (not at all) | 86 | 59.3 | 92 | 62.6 | 32 | 21.8 | 48 | 32.2 | 51 | 34.9 | 90 | 62.9 |
| 2 | 24 | 16.6 | 22 | 15.0 | 11 | 7.5 | 21 | 14.1 | 37 | 25.3 | 18 | 12.6 |
| 3 (somewhat) | 23 | 15.9 | 20 | 13.6 | 33 | 22.5 | 39 | 26.2 | 36 | 24.7 | 27 | 18.9 |
| 4 | 10 | 6.9 | 10 | 6.8 | 33 | 22.5 | 32 | 21.5 | 19 | 13.0 | 5 | 3.5 |
| 5 (very much) | 2 | 1.4 | 3 | 2.0 | 38 | 25.9 | 9 | 6.0 | 3 | 2.1 | 3 | 2.1 |
| Median | 1 | | 1 | | 3 | | 3 | | 2 | | 1 | |
| Mean | 1.7 | | 1.7 | | 3.2 | | 2.6 | | 2.2 | | 1.7 | |
| SD | 1.0 | | 1.1 | | 1.5 | | 1.3 | | 1.1 | | 1.0 | |

**The extent of decreased use of antipsychotics due to the potential adverse effects in the treatment of agitation or psychosis in patients with dementia within the past year (1 = not at all, 3 = somewhat, 5 = very much)** *(continued)*

**21j. OTHER**

| Extent of decreased use | Aripiprazole (n=65) | | Haloperidol (n=65) | | Olanzapine (n=62) | | Quetiapine (n=63) | | Risperidone (n=63) | | Ziprasidone (n=60) | |
|---|---|---|---|---|---|---|---|---|---|---|---|---|
| | No. | % | No. | % | No. | % | No. | % | No. | % | No. | % |
| 1 (not at all) | 42 | 64.6 | 43 | 65.2 | 35 | 56.5 | 31 | 49.2 | 37 | 58.7 | 37 | 61.7 |
| 2 | 4 | 6.2 | 4 | 6.1 | 5 | 8.1 | 2 | 3.2 | 9 | 14.3 | 7 | 11.7 |
| 3 (somewhat) | 11 | 16.9 | 6 | 9.1 | 10 | 16.1 | 15 | 23.8 | 9 | 14.3 | 7 | 11.7 |
| 4 | 4 | 6.2 | 4 | 6.1 | 4 | 6.5 | 6 | 9.5 | 4 | 6.4 | 3 | 5.0 |
| 5 (very much) | 4 | 6.2 | 9 | 13.6 | 8 | 12.9 | 9 | 14.3 | 4 | 6.4 | 6 | 10.0 |
| **Median** | 1 | | 1 | | 1 | | 2 | | 1 | | 1 | |
| **Mean** | 1.8 | | 2.0 | | 2.1 | | 2.4 | | 1.9 | | 1.9 | |
| **SD** | 1.3 | | 1.5 | | 1.5 | | 1.5 | | 1.2 | | 1.4 | |

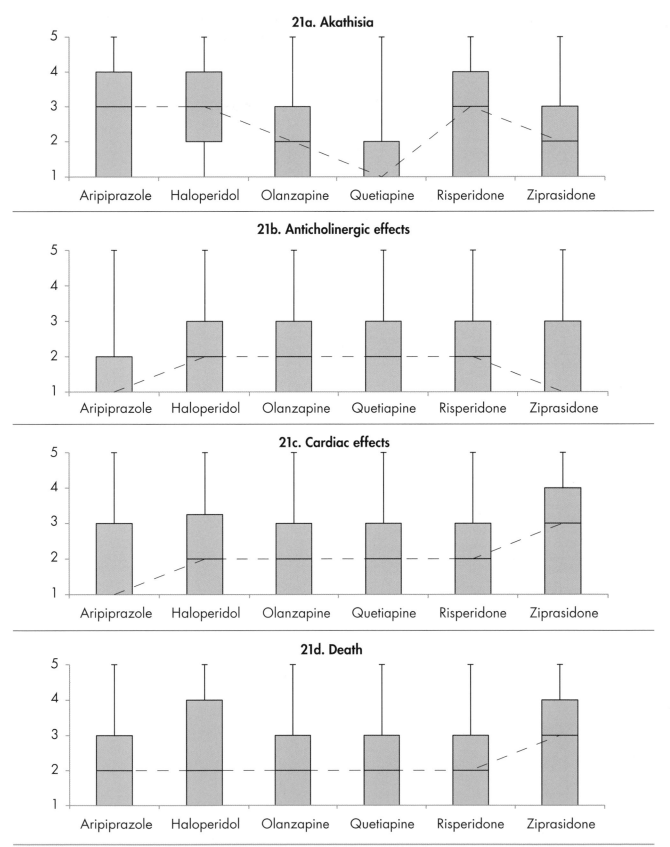

**21a. Akathisia**

**21b. Anticholinergic effects**

**21c. Cardiac effects**

**21d. Death**

**FIGURE B–22.** The extent of decreased use of antipsychotics due to the potential adverse effects in the treatment of agitation or psychosis in patients with dementia within the past year (1 = not at all, 3 = somewhat, 5 = very much).

*Practice Guideline on Use of Antipsychotics to Treat Agitation or Psychosis in Patients With Dementia* **205**

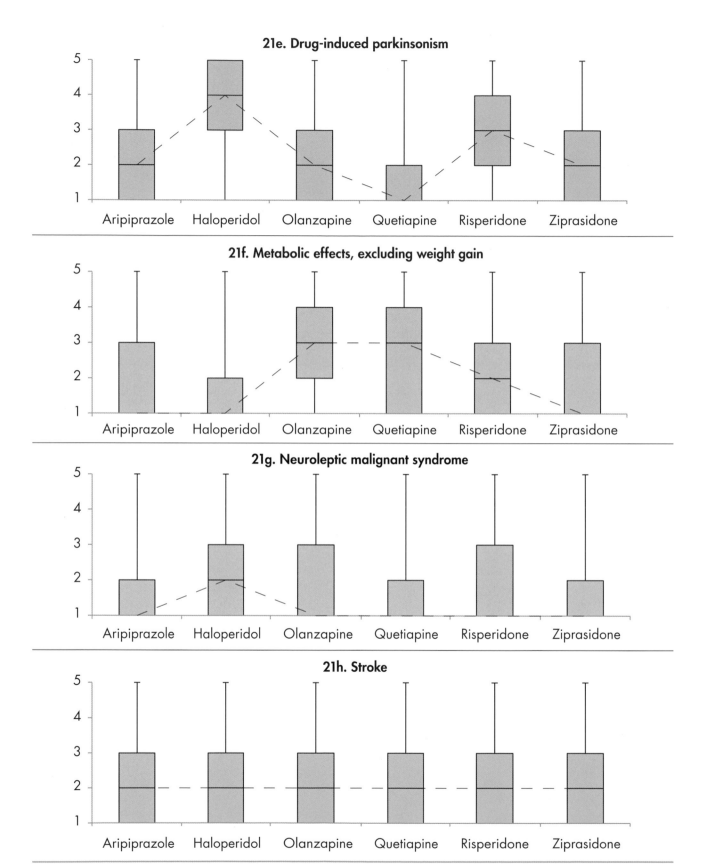

**FIGURE B–22.** The extent of decreased use of antipsychotics due to the potential adverse effects in the treatment of agitation or psychosis in patients with dementia within the past year (1 = not at all, 3 = somewhat, 5 = very much). *(continued)*

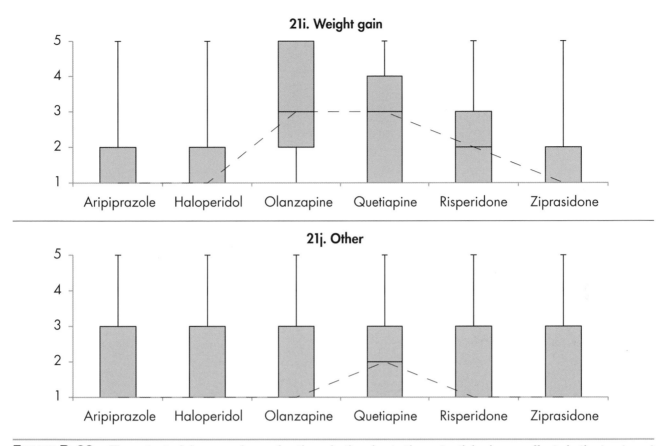

**FIGURE B–22.** The extent of decreased use of antipsychotics due to the potential adverse effects in the treatment of agitation or psychosis in patients with dementia within the past year (1 = not at all, 3 = somewhat, 5 = very much). *(continued)*

**22. Which of the following antipsychotics would you refuse to prescribe to a patient with dementia because of the potential adverse effects? (Check more than one if needed.)**

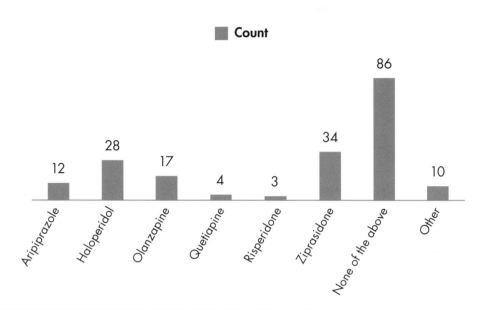

**FIGURE B–23.**  Antipsychotics that experts would refuse to prescribe to a patient with dementia because of the potential adverse effects—checked more than one if needed.

**23. Which of the following prevented you in your own clinical practice from using antipsychotics to treat AGITATION in your patients with dementia WITHIN THE PAST YEAR? (You may select more than one antipsychotic in each row.)**

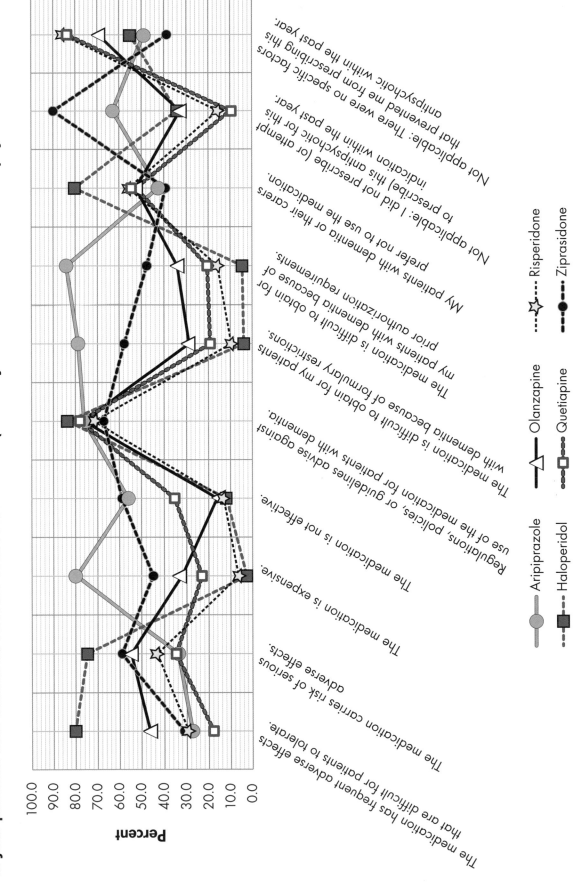

**Figure B–24.** Factors that prevented experts in their own clinical practice from using antipsychotics to treat AGITATION in patients with dementia WITHIN THE PAST YEAR—allowed to select more than one antipsychotic in each factor.

*Practice Guideline on Use of Antipsychotics to Treat Agitation or Psychosis in Patients With Dementia* **209**

**24. Which of the following prevented you in your own clinical practice from using antipsychotics to treat PSYCHOSIS in your patients with dementia WITHIN THE PAST YEAR? (You may select more than one antipsychotic in each row.)**

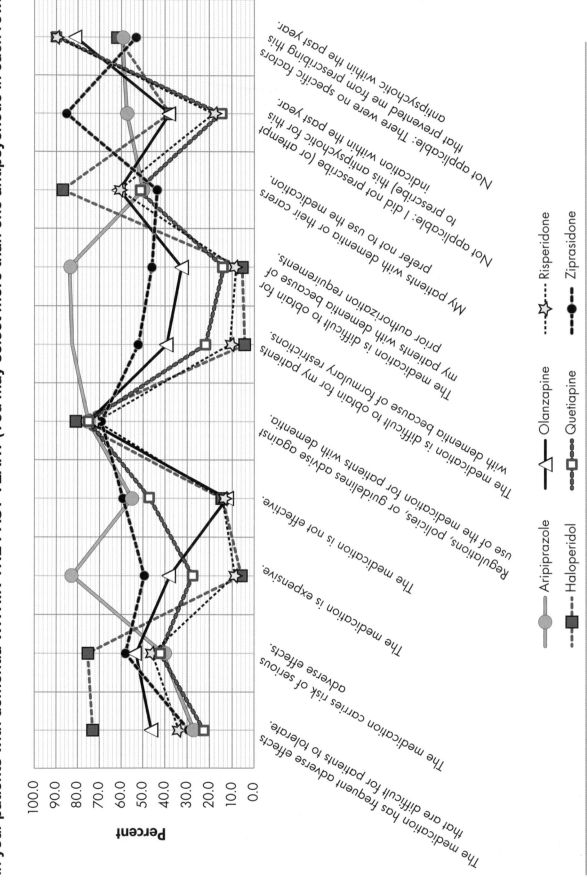

**FIGURE B–25.** Factors that prevented experts in their own clinical practice from using antipsychotics to treat PSYCHOSIS in patients with dementia WITHIN THE PAST YEAR—allowed to select more than one antipsychotic in each factor.

APA Practice Guidelines